Lean Doctors

Best Wishes Lee Anne !

5/21/10

[signature]

Also available from ASQ Quality Press:

Quality Function Deployment and Lean Six Sigma Applications in Public Health
Grace L. Duffy, John W. Moran, and William Riley

The Public Health Quality Improvement Handbook
Ron Bialek, John W. Moran, and Grace L. Duffy

Root Cause Analysis and Improvement in the Healthcare Sector:
A Step-by-Step Guide
Bjørn Andersen, Tom Fagerhaug, and Marti Beltz

Solutions to the Healthcare Quality Crisis: Cases and Examples of
Lean Six Sigma in Healthcare
Soren Bisgaard, editor

On Becoming Exceptional: SSM Health Care's Journey to Baldrige and Beyond
Sister Mary Jean Ryan, FSM

Journey to Excellence: Baldrige Health Care Leaders Speak Out
Kathleen Goonan, editor

A Lean Guide to Transforming Healthcare: How to Implement Lean Principles
in Hospitals, Medical Offices, Clinics, and Other Healthcare Organizations
Thomas G. Zidel

Benchmarking for Hospitals: Achieving Best-in-Class Performance without
Having to Reinvent the Wheel
Victor Sower, Jo Ann Duffy, and Gerald Kohers

Lean-Six Sigma for Healthcare, Second Edition: A Senior Leader Guide to
Improving Cost and Throughput
Greg Butler, Chip Caldwell, and Nancy Poston

Lean Six Sigma for the Healthcare Practice: A Pocket Guide
Roderick A. Munro

Lean for Service Organizations and Offices: A Holistic Approach for
Achieving Operational Excellence and Improvements
Debashis Sarkar

To request a complimentary catalog of ASQ Quality Press publications, call
800-248-1946, or visit our Web site at http://www.asq.org/quality-press.

Lean Doctors

A Bold and Practical Guide to Using Lean Principles to Transform Healthcare Systems, One Doctor at a Time

Aneesh Suneja with Carolyn Suneja

ASQ Quality Press
Milwaukee, Wisconsin

American Society for Quality, Quality Press, Milwaukee, WI 53203
© 2010 by ASQ
All rights reserved. Published 2010.
Printed in the United States of America.

16   15   14   13   12   11   10   5   4   3   2   1

Library of Congress Cataloging-in-Publication Data

Suneja, Aneesh, 1968-
Lean doctors: a bold and practical guide to using lean principles to transform
healthcare systems, one doctor at a time / Aneesh Suneja with Carolyn Suneja.
    p.; cm.
Includes bibliographical references and index.
ISBN 978-0-87389-785-3 (alk. paper)
1. Medical offices – Planning. 2. Lean manufacturing. I. Suneja, Carolyn, 1968-
II. American Society for Quality. III. Title.
[DNLM: 1. Professional Practice – organization & administration. 2. Delivery of
Health Care – organization & administration. 3. Efficiency, Organizational.
4. Physician-Patient Relations. W 87 S958L 2010]
R728.S93 2010
610.68–dc22
                                    2010002393

Publisher: William A. Tony
Acquisitions Editor: Matt T. Meinholz
Project Editor: Paul O'Mara
Production Administrator: Randall Benson

ASQ Mission: The American Society for Quality advances individual,
organizational, and community excellence worldwide through learning, quality
improvement, and knowledge exchange.

Attention Bookstores, Wholesalers, Schools, and Corporations: ASQ Quality
Press books, video, audio, and software are available at quantity discounts with
bulk purchases for business, educational, or instructional use. For information,
please contact ASQ Quality Press at 800-248-1946, or write to ASQ Quality Press,
P.O. Box 3005, Milwaukee, WI 53201-3005.

To place orders or to request ASQ membership information, call 800-248-1946.
Visit our Web site at www.asq.org / quality-press.

♾ Printed on acid-free paper

Quality Press
600 N. Plankinton Avenue
Milwaukee, Wisconsin 53203
Call toll free 800-248-1946
Fax 414-272-1734
www.asq.org
http://www.asq.org/quality-press
http://standardsgroup.asq.org
E-mail: authors@asq.org

Dedication

This book is dedicated with gratitude to
Ms. Terry Schwartz, Orthopedic Program Administrator
for Children's Hospital of Wisconsin.

Contents

List of Figures and Tables

Foreword

I first met Aneesh Suneja about four years ago when he was brought to Children's Hospital of Wisconsin to find ways we might be able to put Lean manufacturing principles to work here. He began sharing excellent thoughts about using Lean to eliminate waste and improve our processes. I immediately realized these ideas held great promise. Although I was not exactly sure how we'd be able to apply manufacturing principles to healthcare, I was curious and soon, I was impressed.

Aneesh is someone who is able to give very clear explanations of rather complicated principles. His methodology is based upon sound principles and data—data that physicians are drawn to. He looks to understand why processes were put in place or why things were done a certain way and then works to support that process. He does not attempt to simply superimpose a single solution onto all problems.

You'll find he takes this same approach throughout this book. He explains the technical principles of Lean in a very easy-to-understand and approachable way. Not only does he truly understand Lean, he understands healthcare. Because of this he is able to not only explain the principles themselves, but also provide very clear, specific ways to adapt and apply these principles to hospitals, clinics, and other healthcare settings. These principles work. We've seen it for ourselves at Children's Hospital of Wisconsin. And I'm confident they'll work in your healthcare setting as well.

I will, however, offer one word of caution: this approach is not a quick fix. You will need to engage in a thoughtful and thorough process. You'll need to be open to looking at things differently, to trying a new approach. You shouldn't expect instantaneous results, and you shouldn't expect that you'll be able to have the same success in every area where you implement Lean. But this is not about fixing it quickly. It's about fixing it correctly.

My hope is that within healthcare we'll be able to continue to look outside of the traditional healthcare environment for solutions—to look to manufacturing and other areas for solid, proven ideas that work. I hope that we'll be open-minded, and able to value and embrace principles like Lean in order to provide patients with the safest, highest-quality, and most efficient care. That, after all, is why we all are engaged in constantly improving.

Michael F. Gutzeit, M.D.
Chief Medical Officer and Vice President of Quality
Children's Hospital of Wisconsin

Acknowledgments

We would like to thank those who encouraged us to complete this book, and who offered their expertise and feedback during the writing process: Dr. Ramesh Sachdeva, Dr. Channing Tassone, Dr. Michael Gutzeit, Dr. Jeffrey Schwab, Dr. Kevin Walter, Dr. Tom Rice, Dr. Theresa Mikhailov, Mr. Larry Duncan, Ms. Lee Anne Eddy, Ms. Maryanne Kessel, Ms. Stephanie Lenzner, Ms. Allison Duey-Holtz, Ms. Sara Collins, Ms. Tracie Brasch, Ms. Lori Seubert, Ms. Beth Wahlquist, and Ms. Julie Pedretti, along with the entire staff at the Orthopedic Center of Children's Hospital of Wisconsin.

Many thanks to Lisa Holewa, writer, friend and cheerleader, whose enthusiasm and journalistic instincts were indispensable in the writing of this book. And finally, thanks to our parents and our three daughters—Jaya, Mya and Emma—for their patience and support.

Introduction

I came to healthcare after spending a decade applying Lean manufacturing principles in slightly more traditional settings, transforming the processes used to make everything from yachts and military helicopters to the paint you use on your living room walls. In this way, I came to realize that Lean, when applied deeply and cohesively, could transform *any* process.

When I began translating Lean to healthcare, I started at the Orthopedic Center of Children's Hospital of Wisconsin. The world of pediatric medicine is set in a fragile, human, and emotional environment, perhaps the place most unlike an automotive assembly line that you could imagine. At the Orthopedic Center, for example, children's bones are mended and surgeons work to abate the effects of scoliosis that twists young spines. So much depends upon perception, intuition, and skill.

Clearly, this is a place where results matter. And so I will begin by sharing the numbers.

As a direct result of our Lean transformation, the Orthopedic Center increased its "fractures patient volume" (or, more simply, the number of patients seen with bone fractures) by 25 percent, in the same amount of time, with the same number of staff—and using 25 percent fewer exam rooms. The important healthcare measure of "time to next appointment" has been reduced by more than 33 percent (from three weeks to less than two weeks). Weekly access for new fracture patients increased by 20 percent. And the clinic has reduced patient wait times by more than 70 percent.

Most importantly, this was achieved with a focus clearly set on quality patient care. The interaction between the doctor and patient in the exam room was left completely untouched, with all the other changes designed to improve the quality and result of that interaction.

Again, look to the numbers: the clinic has achieved instances of 100 percent patient satisfaction, which is remarkable. Staff satisfaction scores have soared as well, often nearing 99 percent in internal staff satisfaction surveys.

As you consider undergoing a Lean transformation process at your own practice or clinic (or hospital or larger healthcare setting), you might think that a minute shaved off here and a minute saved there does not seem worth much. Change is difficult, time-consuming, and cumbersome. So why would you literally analyze every step a nurse takes? Why take the time to have technicians or nurse practitioners describe in detail the reality of their jobs, when you need them to simply get the work done?

Why? Because it works. Tell a doctor that he can see the same number of patients, offering the same high quality and personal care, and have an extra 90 minutes at the end of his clinic day—and that means something. Tell the staff that they can look forward to actually ending on time, with satisfied patients, no backlog, and having focused their attention completely on quality patient care—and they will listen.

There are, of course, many compelling reasons to begin a Lean transformation process, but considering the numbers is always a good place to begin. Imagine your clinic or practice or hospital could do 25 percent more with exactly the same resources, simply by rethinking its processes. That's what Lean is all about.

WHAT INEFFICIENCY IN HEALTHCARE SETTINGS MEANS FOR PATIENTS

I'd like to shift focus for a moment from the doctors, nurses, and healthcare executives to the patients they serve. Rather than discussing data, here I'm going to share a simple story.

Several years ago, my four-year-old daughter tripped in the grass and landed hard on her arm. As I watched her elbow quickly swell and change color, my heart sped with worry. Where was the nearest emergency room? Could I get her buckled into her booster seat in the car without further hurting her? How would I calm her?

The ensuing emergency room visit was an experience similar to one most parents face at some point. We arrived quickly and were able to get into an exam room after a short wait in a triage area. But then things slowed. The process of getting her seen by a physician and into a temporary splint took nearly three hours. Then we waited another 90 minutes for an orthopedic surgeon to return a call about the diagnosis, before the emergency room doctor simply sent us home for the night. We would see the surgeon tomorrow.

At the orthopedic clinic the next day, I witnessed what happens when well-intentioned people work like crazy in an inefficient system. Certainly no one meant to be inefficient. Each individual person did his or her job well—from the pleasant person at the front desk to the empathetic casting technician who gave my daughter her choice of glitter colors. But no one was responsible for getting us in and out quickly with the care we needed. The system almost seemed *designed* to make patients wait. We waited to get into an exam room. We waited to get an x-ray. We waited to get a diagnosis. We waited to get a cast. And we waited to get the educational materials we needed. We took these wait times for granted; after all, this was a busy clinic and the staff was really moving—harried, even.

But, as someone who had spent his career analyzing how processes work and where they break down, I knew that these wait times had both deeper roots and more significance than the obvious busy-ness of the clinic. For starters, the long wait times meant that there was more opportunity for things to go wrong. On an entirely different level, the long wait times meant that the clinic was not operating as efficiently as it could—that basic improvements could be made to bolster communication, align processes, and impact the quality of patient care.

Like any other parent, of course, I also could simply sense that despite all that activity and hurrying around on the part of the staff, a fundamental coordination was lacking. Who was driving this bus? We left the clinic feeling a bit unsettled and uncertain.

This story of my daughter's broken arm and her treatment at the clinic is in no way unique; in fact, it is a pretty run-of-the mill experience. What makes the story just a bit different is, as you may have guessed, that I ended up in that same clinic a few months later—this time as a consultant hired to use the Lean manufacturing principles pioneered by Toyota to eliminate waste and improve efficiency.

(Throughout this book, I'm going to assume that you have a fundamental knowledge of Lean, and that you already know a bit about its history, principles, and methods. This way, I can focus more directly on how to successfully translate the processes to the healthcare environment. If you're not confident that you already have a solid grasp on the principles, or if you'd like to learn more about the origins and evolution of Lean, take a look at the overview in the appendix. There, you'll also find a glossary of terms and resources for learning more about implementing the principles. I'm also providing an overview of my own experience and how I've applied the principles to a variety of different industries, summarizing what I learned each step of the way. Begin with the appendix if you'd like any of this background.)

Of course, it's important to note that Children's Hospital of Wisconsin already had various quality improvement programs in place before we began our work at the Orthopedic Center. Although some healthcare organizations have taken an "all-or-none" approach to Lean, the truth is that it also can work in conjunction with other quality programs. I'll discuss that in more detail as we continue.

Clinics—from the walk-in clinic at the local drugstore staffed by a nurse practitioner to a bustling Orthopedic Center in a hospital setting—provide Americans with a majority of their healthcare. There are more than 25,000 clinics in the United States *(2002 Economic Census)*, providing care in an estimated 500 million visits per year *(Kaiser Family Foundation)*.

These clinics represent a huge first-step opportunity for improvement in healthcare. They are led by a physician and a small team of providers who create their own processes and have some level of control over how those processes operate—something known as a "healthcare microsystem." The individual physician sets the tone for the clinic through her scheduling preferences and manner of seeing patients. As such, that physician has the ability to change and improve the clinic's processes in a tangible and direct way.

WHY APPLY LEAN TO HEALTHCARE SETTINGS?

Healthcare reform is front and center in the American political debate, and it is a topic that directly affects the lives of countless Americans. It seems no matter what you read, the same statistics resurface: healthcare spending was $2.2 trillion in 2007, or more than 16 percent of the Gross Domestic Product. Eighty-seven million people went without health insurance at some point during 2007 and 2008. Costs are projected to rise to 25 percent of the GDP by 2025. The United States spends nearly twice as much on healthcare as other developed countries, but achieves no better health outcomes than most of those nations, leading analysts to label the U.S. system as inefficient.

Although the complex underlying causes of inefficiency in the U.S. healthcare system are widely debated, it is much harder to find reports offering solutions of any kind. So the dedicated doctors, nurses, and providers in the trenches—like the cast tech with her red glitter for a four-year-old with a broken arm—are caught in the eye of the storm. Not surprisingly, they find themselves overwhelmed at the magnitude of change that must occur, frustrated by their own lack of empowerment to make any change happen, and simply too busy providing care to step back and evaluate the processes they operate.

This dynamic is exactly what I found when I began working with Children's Hospital in 2005, starting in the Orthopedic Center and its operating room. (I moved on to apply Lean at Children's in the Neurology clinic, the Herma Heart center, the Emergency Department, the operating rooms, and the Intensive Care Unit, and I will touch upon some ways we translated the principles to those environments. But since our initial work was in Orthopedics, where the entire clinic has now undergone the Lean transformation and we already have the data detailing the impact of our changes, this case study will focus on that area.)

At the Orthopedic Center, I found talented, dedicated people who sincerely wanted to make a meaningful difference in the lives of their young patients and their families. This desire was precisely why they went into the pediatric healthcare field. And yet I found that their clinic processes—how the clinic was run—had migrated away from the original patient focus. Layers of handoffs and complications had been created, in large part because of a traditional department structure (in which, for example, "Radiology" was a separate department from "Orthopedics").

I also found inspired leadership ready to take on bold new change, willing to question and challenge the "how" and "why" of their clinic processes. And so my work with the Orthopedic team began as a bit of an experiment, based on a hunch that the principles of Lean could be employed in healthcare far beyond the then-emerging model of simply organizing supply carts and using pull systems for ordering forms.

As I mentioned, my experience over the previous decade implementing Lean in manufacturing industries had proven to me that the principles of Lean could transform *any* value stream if applied deeply and as a cohesive whole. But the literature in healthcare at the time was filled with superficial techniques that circled around—but did not touch—the one critical lynchpin in the entire system: the physician.

Of course, there are a lot of reasons to leave physicians and their work alone. First and most importantly, physicians are highly educated professionals who spend years gaining the knowledge and experience needed to walk into an exam room and provide an accurate diagnosis and care plan. Rightly, few quality improvement efforts want to intrude upon the sanctity of the physician-patient consultation.

In addition, physicians often report through separate lines of authority than other staff at the clinic, making it difficult to drive improvements that affect everyone. Finally, there is simply the fact that the person being called "doctor" has a certain aura and authority that by itself creates distance between that physician and the rest of the staff. Where there are strong personalities and preferences about how clinic processes operate, the rest of the staff learns to work around the physician. And even in environments where the physician and his staff are on the same team, most times the staff will simply do what they perceive the doctor wants without questioning the underlying process.

As a result, quality improvement initiatives often focus on the roles nurses, physician assistants, clinic assistants, and others play—in isolation from the physician. Unfortunately, this leaves the team to make changes that may be beneficial, but are nonetheless peripheral to the "meat and potatoes" of the clinic's work. No matter how efficiently a patient is checked in or roomed, if the physician is reviewing billing documents or dictating when she should be in the exam room, the clinic comes to a halt.

STRATEGIC DECISIONS THAT MADE OUR LEAN TRANSFORMATION WORK

At the outset, I made two strategic decisions that became formative in the creation of our Lean transformation process for healthcare settings: first, to work with one physician at a time—with the emphasis both on *one* and *physician*; and second, to focus exclusively on patient wait times.

The decision to work with one physician at a time meant that the physician would be the one leading the area's improvement efforts. In this case, choosing that physician was a crucial step in beginning our process. The physician had to have the potential to be a champion for Lean; he had to be open to change and value quality improvement. The physician and his team of nurses, technicians, and administrative support would work together to analyze their current state and participate in a series of workshops to make meaningful and lasting change.

There are several ways in which Lean solutions are being used and tested in healthcare. This includes providing Lean awareness training for the entire staff, or creating value stream maps to identify projects across the board. It includes Kaizen events focused on prioritized problems, or implementing one Lean tool at a time—and various hybrids of all of these approaches.

In many implementations, Lean efforts begin with training—often a *lot* of training delivered broadly across the healthcare organization—and then move on to implementing a pilot project or two system-wide. The training is done under the premise that people must be made aware of what the Lean effort is all about before they can participate in it. However, I have found that the traditional training-based approach is flawed in several fundamental ways.

First, it is a *push* system. In Lean parlance, a push system is one in which a product is moved to the next step in the process whether or not that step is ready for it. When training is pushed onto an audience, the investment of time and money made in that training is likely to be lost as people have no immediate opportunity to use what they are learning. They become frustrated or simply forget what they heard. Ideally, improvement initiatives and their associated training should be "pulled" by the workforce so that the methodologies and the tools can be quickly applied and do not fall on deaf ears.

Second, the training-then-pilot-projects approach often *stays* very superficial, simply because its scope is too broad. Many healthcare organizations opt to conduct 5S workshops in many areas, for example, choosing to implement one tool everywhere rather than a true Lean system in one place. Others might create rolling supply carts everywhere in an attempt to implement the Lean principle of minimal motion. Others might implement Standard Work, Error-Proofing, or Visual Controls. It does not matter what the particular Lean tool is. In my experience, one tool applied broadly across the healthcare organization will never yield results to equal the entire Lean system applied thoroughly in one physician's clinic.

My final reason for the one-doctor-at-a-time approach is that broad training-based Lean implementations too often get a reputation for being the "flavor of the month" because they lack sustainable results. It is a truth of the business world, no matter the industry, that what gets results gets paid for. Large training initiatives are expensive. Widespread one-tool roll-outs are expensive. If the only resulting metric is the number of people trained or the number of rapid improvement workshops held, that improvement initiative will not withstand the scrutiny of cost-conscious healthcare executives. In order to last long enough to have a real impact on the healthcare delivery system, improvement initiatives must be measured in business metrics such as revenue, cost avoidance, and outcomes.

The approach I took of implementing Lean one physician at a time also had the benefit of allowing small teams of people to conduct quick experiments in their process and get immediate feedback. It allowed for great nimbleness and focus in the improvement work that a larger rollout would have precluded based on the sheer number of people involved. And it allowed the other physicians running clinics in Orthopedics to see the target team's difference and wonder, for example, why that doctor's team got to go home on time or why their working environment seemed less stressful. As the culture of the Lean target clinic transformed, other physicians began to *pull* the improvement process, ensuring that money invested in Lean work was being spent where it had the best chance of being met with motivation and enthusiasm.

The one-doctor-at-a-time approach also resonated with healthcare professionals who were used to large quality improvement initiatives imposed upon them by what they perceived to be a less-than-insightful management structure. Focusing not just on one area or specialty, but on one physician within that area, gave the team a unique opportunity to have their opinions heard and their specific issues addressed. Eventually the Lean transformation reached as many people and areas within the organization as it would have if we had begun with large-scale training, but it reached them in a way that made them want to respond and engage.

The second strategic decision was to focus on patient wait times as the metric driving the improvement efforts. Why wait times? Why not errors, or patient satisfaction, or staff turnover? Why not a scorecard of metrics that would measure a laundry list of performance indicators?

Lean is a science for creating flow in a system—whether of a physical product or of a service. In healthcare, this would mean that we aim to create patient flow, without wait times, through any given area. As we focused on patient wait times in the clinic we found that no other metric brought the varied root causes of inefficiency so clearly into focus. When patients were moving through the process promptly, a lot of things were going right. However, when patients waited in the exam rooms or waiting rooms or at supplying processes, then any one of a great number of things could be going wrong. (If, for example, patients are waiting outside of radiology in the Orthopedic Center, it could be because the scheduling template does not provide a level schedule, or that radiology is understaffed or equipment is broken, or because communication about patient status broke down and no one knows where those patients are.)

Long wait times for patients also indicate that resources in the clinic are being wasted. If a patient is in the exam room, waiting for service, it means that room is tied up and not available for the next patient. It means that staff members may make several non-value added trips around the clinic, trying to get the physician to see the patient or trying to explain the reasons for delay to the patient family. The quality of care can suffer if the physician is moving from one patient to another in a chaotic manner. This experience may also turn into a patient complaint and consume more valuable resources in the hospital.

I'll use my earlier story again as an example. Despite the fact that my daughter and I had a scheduled appointment time, we waited nearly 20 minutes to get into a cast room. Did that wait time indicate that the cast technician did not know we were there? Or that the scheduling template had placed too many new patients in a row for the cast staff to handle? Focusing on wait times forces the project team to uncover those varied root causes and implement changes to fix them one at a time. Further, uncovering those causes also leads to discovering a long chain of inefficiencies, handoffs, and errors that require the project team to collaborate with other functions within the healthcare system. So, asking the question, "Why did the clinic run over 45 minutes tonight?" can result in improvements involving not only the clinic staff, but the scheduling team and support functions as well.

THE IMPORTANCE OF TAKING A VALUE STREAM APPROACH

These two ideas—working with one physician at a time and focusing on patient wait times—are the key differentiators for the process described in this book. In order to put these ideas into action, a clinic or practice has to take a "value stream approach" to Lean in healthcare. Taking a value stream approach simply means looking at the big picture—the entire process of providing care—from the patient's perspective. There is no room for isolated "Lean projects" in this approach. (Projects are often intended to implement a particular tool of Lean, like 5S or visual communication, but because they are disconnected from a larger system perspective, the results that can be achieved are very limited.)

In keeping with that patient-centered value stream approach, we've developed six success steps to implementing Lean in any healthcare environment that I'd like to introduce now. These steps support the underlying principles of making change one physician at a time and focusing on patient wait times. Each step builds upon the previous step in the Lean transformation process. Like the underlying principles, they will be described in greater detail throughout this book. Here is a quick summary:

1. *Create physician flow:* This centers on the idea of the physician as a "shared resource"—a pacemaker in the process—who should never have down time due to missing information or lack of clear priorities. Everything except the physician's consultation with the patient is essentially changeover and should be done as efficiently as possible to set the doctor up for the best possible patient interaction.

2. *Support physician value-added time:* In order for the physician to maintain a state of flow and not experience undue downtime, she needs a high level of coordination of clinic processes. This step calls for the creation of a team leader position, whose primary responsibility is to make sure the doctor's time is used effectively. The team leader is usually a nurse who has leadership potential; the duties include tracking the status of each patient and "driving the bus" to direct the clinic.

3. *Visually communicate patient status:* Visual communication is the Lean concept of using visible markers, signals, and signs to communicate the status of a given process so that anyone walking into the work environment can tell what's in process, what's working, and where the problems are. With this step, I describe a seemingly simple, powerful tool in the clinic setting: the Patient Status Whiteboard.

4. *Standardize everyone's work:* Standard work is a tool of Lean that provides process stability and a mechanism for formal process improvement. In this step the care team creates standard work for their processes to find immediate improvement opportunities, achieve predictable outcomes, and clarify their roles in the care process. Creating standard work also formalizes changes made so far and helps the Lean system become an integral part of the practice's culture.

5. *Lay out the clinic for minimal motion:* This step focuses on examining how to change the physical layout of a clinic or other healthcare environment to improve patient flow and staff communication. It uses the tools of spaghetti mapping and 5S to look at individual workstations, and discusses the flow of care and communication throughout the clinic. Some of the Lean improvements discussed here are simple ones: creating supply and material carts, moving commonly used forms and supplies inside the exam rooms, organizing paperwork at the front desk, and establishing "pull" by creating a kanban card system. Architectural improvements, such as U-shaped cell designs, help develop an enhanced team space to improve patient safety, staff communication, and patient handoffs.

6. *Change the care delivery model:* This means rethinking the clinic processes to focus relentlessly on patient flow. The idea of focusing on flow is central to Lean, because organizing work in departments simply does not work. Support departments—such as radiology, casting, physical therapy, labs, echo, and pharmacy—should be rethought and broken into decentralized mini-departments, where feasible. The previous steps—managing the physician's time, visually controlling patient status, standardizing the individual tasks in the care process—lay a stable foundation so that larger process changes do not create chaos.

The results of this approach are impressive, even more so because they are sustainable. As I mentioned earlier, the Orthopedic Center reduced patient wait times by more than 70 percent, indicating that a great many things now are indeed going right. They can see 25 percent more patients in less space, and have achieved instances of 100 percent patient satisfaction scores. Staff satisfaction scores have improved by more than 25 percent, and health professionals from other areas have actually requested moves into the clinics where the Lean transformation has occurred. (See Table I.1.)

It's important to note that it's not just the processes that have changed. With the creation of team leaders, nurses who are directly responsible for the flow of patients through the clinic, the organizational structure has changed to support the Lean vision. Further, the management structure has changed. Gone are the days of contentious relationships between physicians and managers; the performance data collected by the team and shared with management and physicians allows for better decision making and fundamentally changes how patient-centered issues get resolved. Physicians and managers work collaboratively because they are aligned around patient needs, analyze the same data, and play clearly defined roles.

Table I.1 Dr. Tassone Fractures Clinic results.

Category	Before	After	Metric	% Change
Patient Volumes (4-hour clinic)	40	50	Number of Patients	Up 25%
Space	6	4.5	Number of Exam Rooms	Down 25%
Space Utilization* (PA clinic created)	0	6	Number of Patients	Up 100%
Patient Wait Times	38	11	Minutes from Door to Provider	Down 71%

A Physician's Assistant clinic (during Dr. Tassone's clinic) opened up in the freed-up space.

This book is the result of my belief in this process. These Lean principles and success steps work. They work in clinics from orthopedics to neurology to cardiac care—the specialty doesn't matter. They work in small practices and large hospital settings. Lean methodology provides the tools to address the frustrations patients and doctors experience in the clinic process.

The Orthopedic Center at Children's Hospital of Wisconsin is now a model of efficiency and patient satisfaction, one that hospital executives and quality-minded professionals routinely tour to glimpse these principles in action. Physicians have in hand all the information they need to see patients before they walk in the room. They are supported by a team that understands what must happen next and how to make it happen efficiently. Patients spend less time in the clinic, yet more time with their doctor. The process moves along smoothly, the clinic day ends on time, and the staff reports less stress. Best of all, the team has sharpened its focus on the patient, providing top quality care—and still has time for glitter.

A recent opinion piece in the *New England Journal of Medicine* urges physicians to take the lead in improving care processes: "Healthcare microsystems are famously unreliable, variable in costs, and often unsafe. Physicians, through their participation in quality-improvement initiatives in their practices and hospitals, can and should lead the needed changes in the systems of care in which they work, to make them safer, more reliable, more patient-centered, and more affordable."

Lean methodology provides the tools to address the frustrations patients and doctors alike experience in the healthcare setting. What is needed is for physicians to drive the transformation.

You can find one physician (or be that physician) who can champion the Lean transformation for the front line in your clinic or practice. Take a value stream perspective and evaluate the current state from the patient's point of view. Align the team around the patient so that the team's interactions are focused on that common goal instead of on personalities and turf wars. Then explore the principles and steps presented in this book, one at a time, and let your Lean transformation begin.

Two Strategic Decisions

1

Begin One Doctor
at a Time

L et's step back for a moment and imagine you're about to run your
first marathon. The starting gun cracks and you take off at a sprint,
quickly covering the first stretch. You're ahead of the pack. Your
numbers look great. And so you push on, full speed ahead.

But no matter how determined you are, no matter how strong, the
truth is you'll soon find yourself out of breath, exhausted and, worst of
all, nowhere near the finish line. So, at maybe the two-mile mark, you
drop out. And you darkly remind yourself: *"I didn't think I could run a
marathon, anyway."*

Described in these terms, it's clear you set yourself up for failure,
that your strategy determined the outcome before you took your first
step. Yet, I'd argue that this is exactly the approach too many healthcare
organizations take when undertaking quality improvement initiatives.
More specifically, it's the model commonly advocated for Lean transformation processes in healthcare.

The approach goes something like this: Bring your entire healthcare
group together for a series of seminars and training sessions. Then
blanket the place with changes that you label "Lean initiatives," perhaps
setting up supply carts and moving them closer to examination rooms,
or organizing and cleaning out supply rooms and storage, maybe
eliminating a layer of paperwork that is deemed wasteful. The result:
lots of time and money spent on lots of people, with lots of workers and
managers left dealing with changes they may not have initiated and don't
truly understand how to sustain.

My work implementing Lean both in manufacturing and healthcare
settings has convinced me that an approach like this is no better than
taking off for your first marathon at a sprint, covering some ground
quickly, but ultimately getting nowhere.

Even worse, it's my belief that these initiatives, though labeled
"Lean," aren't a true interpretation of the process, which is more truly
hallmarked by a bottom-up (rather than top-down) approach. Lean is

defined by a sense of "pull" rather than "push"—an approach where the people who know and understand the processes (the people who actually do the work) are the ones solidly behind the changes. In order to make this happen, you need a better plan than overwhelming people with training and dictating superficial changes.

It's important to recognize that your goal is not to sprint through a mile or two, amassing impressive numbers but ultimately failing. Instead, you should start by recognizing that a true Lean transformation, like a marathon, requires strength, stamina, and perhaps most importantly, an effective strategy.

VENTURING INTO DEEP WATER (ONE DOCTOR AT A TIME)

I'm going to switch metaphors and say that a true Lean transformation process is not about the river that's a mile wide and an inch deep. A true Lean transformation goes deep into the culture of the clinic or practice. It's not about blanketing an organization with widespread but ultimately shallow training or changes. In order to successfully and truly implement Lean in the healthcare setting, you must venture into the deep water. This is why I take a different approach to implementing Lean, beginning one doctor at a time.

(It's important to note here that in large organizations, this approach does not have to be taken quite so literally. With the proper resources, it can be adapted, for example, to mean one department at a time, or one doctor in each department at a time. However, the idea is to transform one area before moving on to another—to make true and deep changes that take hold and then allow the changes to migrate naturally as word of their success spreads.)

In my approach, the doctor and his team (rather than the entire organization) receive the training and information they need to begin making major changes to the processes they operate. They receive it just hours before they will begin using it. There is no waste in the delivery of information.

As the physician team works to evaluate its processes and make changes, a couple of very powerful things begin to happen.

- First, the team is forced to improve its communication and dynamics. With time, the very culture of that team changes to include norms such as conducting quick experiments to solve problems in real time, focusing on performance goals rather than interpersonal dramas, and continually discussing ways to make the process more efficient and more effective.

- Second, word of the team's transformation spreads in the healthcare organization. In the clinic setting, for example, other physicians and nurses hear of the improved performance and work environment and want to be the next Lean project. As more physician teams take on the Lean work with the same approach, the success continues to build demand. Essentially the Lean work is pulled by the physicians and nurses in the organization, and the knowledge and expertise are replicated.

The approach reaches the same number of people in the organization as does a more common mass-training approach. However, it reaches those people in a fundamentally different way. Rather than training up front and making changes later, teams make significant changes faster and gain the knowledge they need along the way. The engagements offer meaningful, patient-centered results because they make meaningful, patient-centered changes to the way the care delivery system operates.

Before going into more detail about how to implement this one-doctor-at-a-time approach, I want to talk a bit more about the realities of quality improvement initiatives in the healthcare setting, why these efforts often meet resistance, and how and why Lean can be different—leading the way to true and sustainable change that makes a real difference.

As we continue examining how the Orthopedic Center at Children's Hospital of Wisconsin underwent its Lean transformation, allow me to introduce the some of the visionaries in our case study:

- **Ramesh Sachdeva, MD, PhD, MBA, JD** is the corporate vice president and chief quality officer at Children's Hospital and Health System. He is the person who spearheaded the Lean quality improvement efforts at Children's, and the executive responsible for quality improvement programs throughout the organization.

- **Larry Duncan** is the corporate vice president of regional services for Children's Hospital and Health Systems. He was the vice president of ambulatory and diagnostics—overseeing Orthopedics, among other departments, at the time we began our Lean transformation in the Orthopedic Center.

- **Lee Anne Eddy** is the vice president of ambulatory and diagnostic services for Children's Hospital of Wisconsin. She was the director over several areas, including Orthopedics, when we began our work.

(continued)

- **J. Channing Tassone, MD** is an associate professor of Pediatric Orthopedics at the Medical College of Wisconsin. He is an orthopedic surgeon who was our Lean champion in the department and his practice is where we began experimenting with Lean changes.

- **Terry Schwartz** is the program administrator at the Orthopedic Center. She is the administrator I worked with most directly in implementing the Lean changes in the fractures clinic.

- **Stephanie Lenzner, MSHA, MBA** is the director of Quality Data Management at Children's Hospital and Health System. She was our liaison between the Quality Data Management department (which tracks outcomes) and the clinic during our Lean transformation in the Orthopedic Center.

- **Tracie A. Brasch, RN, BSN** is a nurse in the Orthopedic Center at Children's Hospital of Wisconsin. She became one of our first Lean team leaders.

- **Lori Seubert, RN, BSN** is a nurse in the Orthopedic Center at Children's Hospital of Wisconsin. She also became one of our Lean team leaders.

- **Allison Duey-Holtz, RN, MSN, CPNP** is a nurse practitioner for Dr. Tassone. She was instrumental in testing various Lean workflow concepts and later led a team of her peers to create Standard Work for patient care.

- **Beth Wahlquist, RN, BSN** is a nurse in the Orthopedic Center at Children's Hospital of Wisconsin. She also became one of our initial Lean team leaders.

- **Amy Ricely** is Dr. Tassone's administrative assistant. Among her many other duties, she is responsible for scheduling surgical patients.

LEAN WORKS ALONGSIDE OTHER QUALITY IMPROVEMENT TOOLS

It's important to note that, while some healthcare systems have made wholesale, sweeping changes and integrated Lean across the entire organization, Lean does not have to be such a daunting all-or-none proposition. In other words, your goal in beginning this process does not have to be to transform *everything* with Lean. There may be places within your healthcare setting that would benefit most from these Lean principles to eliminate waste and improve efficiency. You might already have other quality improvement processes in place, or even an entire quality improvement department. That's all OK. In fact, it's another reason why a one-doctor-at-a-time approach works so well—it offers the flexibility and scope to allow true, deep, and sustainable change in healthcare microsystems.

At Children's, I worked closely with Dr. Ramesh Sachdeva, a practicing physician and corporate vice president who also has an MBA and a PhD in Epidemiology. (He notes that the Lean effort had the complete support of Children's Hospital and Health System executive vice president and chief operating officer Cindy Christensen, adding: "If she were not committed to that extent, I don't know that we could have been as successful.")

Now the chief quality officer for the Children's Health System, Dr. Sachdeva's research is focused on the area of outcomes analysis. He serves as medical director of Quality Initiatives for the American Academy of Pediatrics. He explains that one of the six dimensions of quality in healthcare is efficiency—and importantly, that improving efficiency isn't simply about improving processes and considering the result in isolation from patient care.

"The point is that it's not just the process that has improved," he says. "Improving efficiency is the equivalent of improving quality of care."

However, there are many methods for improving efficiency (and therefore the quality of patient care), and the tool should fit the problem. "When a child or patient comes to see you, you don't just treat everybody with antibiotics," Dr. Sachdeva notes. "You need to be able to match the solution to the situation."

Knowing that we would be strategically applying Lean one doctor at a time, and realizing that the starting point for this project would be critical to its success, the question became: Where do we begin?

The Children's team ultimately made the decision to begin its Lean journey with the Orthopedic Center based on several important factors, each related to the unique character of Lean principles and to the efficiency problems that needed to be resolved. One major reason for choosing Orthopedics was the clinic's leadership, which we'll talk more about later.

Another factor, as Children's corporate vice president Larry Duncan explains, is that the clinic was facing critical issues involving growth and efficiency. Orthopedics was a fast-growing department with ever-increasing numbers of patients. It was also a "land-locked" department without any space for physical expansion in the near future.

"This was a clinic facing growth without a whole lot of other options," Duncan explains. "I don't believe Lean fits everything, that it's the right answer all the time. But it's a tool that's remarkably effective in the right place. And in some ways, we had a sort of 'perfect storm' for Lean in Orthopedics."

Simply put: The Orthopedic Center had to do more, without being given more space. They needed to get more out of what they already had. "We needed to get the wasted time out of the system," says Duncan. "This was really about operational efficiency. If we can eliminate waste, we can grow without more space."

In many ways, the people within the clinic recognized the same truth, perhaps in an even deeper way. "We were willing to give this a try because the clinic was a mess," nurse Tracie Brasch forthrightly explains. "Our volume was going up but our staffing was staying the same. The needs of the patients were the same, but there were more patients. So we said 'Fine. What do we have to lose?'"

Or, as her colleague nurse Lori Seubert recalls: "We weren't taking care of ourselves. We weren't getting lunch. We weren't getting out on time. So we were willing to give something new a try."

OVERCOMING THE "FLAVOR OF THE MONTH" SYNDROME

You should recognize, of course, that this "buy-in" on the part of the staff was a bit reluctant. Everyone involved now admits to having been skeptical. And this is important to remember: One of your biggest roadblocks when beginning a Lean transformation is the very fact that other quality improvement initiatives already have been tried and failed. Workers have heard it all before. They've been there and done that. They know the mantra: "More, better, faster." Too many outsiders have tried before to tell them how to do their jobs, too many "improvement" measures have come and gone.

At Children's, Orthopedic program administrator Terry Schwartz, who ultimately guided our efforts there, describes it as the "flavor of the month" syndrome: you try something out for a week or a couple months, love it briefly, and then move on to the next great thing.

Or, in the words of the Lee Anne Eddy, the hospital vice president overseeing the Orthopedic department (among other departments): "I wasn't familiar with Lean. I worried perhaps it was just the next gimmick. There's always a cycle, always something new to try—the latest book that's out, the latest strategy—and it sometimes seems we always just end up back where we started."

And these comments are from the people at the upper rungs of management, the ones who have say in making the decisions. Imagine the responses from the nurses, the cast technicians, the administrative assistants—the ones on the front lines, responsible for actually making the clinic work.

Tracie Brasch, the Orthopedic Center nurse, can tell you about that response, because she experienced it first-hand upon hearing news of the Lean initiative. As she puts it: "We've done this. We've been there. It just never sticks. Oh my gosh, don't tell me—here's another thing to take me away from patient care."

More succinctly, from a senior Orthopedic surgeon within the clinic: "I expected another exercise in futility."

This is why you should take Lean slowly. Keep the focus firmly on improving patient care, making true and sustainable changes within a small, dynamic, and adaptable group. And move on only as the evidence of your success spreads and people outside of that first group become intrigued. In other words, proceed carefully…one doctor at a time.

MAKING THE CRITICAL DECISIONS THAT WILL DEFINE YOUR SUCCESS

Of course, approaching Lean one doctor at a time means making several critical decisions up front. Those decisions are all about the starting point: Which physician will be the best champion for Lean? Which manager can drive the Lean work forward as a change agent? Selecting the right area, along with the right change agent and Lean champion, can set your Lean work up for success from the very beginning of the project.

Lee Ann Eddy, the vice president who helped decide to start in the Orthopedic Center, describes the process of making this choice based upon evaluating department managers: "What I was looking for was someone who was interested in it immediately. We could make any leader do it, but we wanted a leader who was clearly interested in it. For us, that was the initial hook."

And it so happened that we were extraordinarily fortunate to begin the Lean transformation work with the Orthopedic Center. Terry Schwartz, the program administrator I quoted earlier, not only immediately "raised her hand" to volunteer, but was in several other ways the ideal change agent. She had a long history of involvement in quality initiatives and tools, and had been active with the Institute for Healthcare Improvement (IHI) and other organizations in her career. She had created an atmosphere in the Orthopedic Center that was open to trying new things and looking for ways to improve. For her team to be the first in the hospital to implement Lean seemed like a natural fit.

"We had trust in her," says Lee Anne Eddy, "and she had a track record of being a good leader."

In addition to her expertise managing quality projects, Terry Schwartz also had operational authority in the Orthopedic Center and the ability to make critical decisions about process changes. She understood the operations well enough to help the team implement changes and remove obstacles to the Lean work. She was well-connected in the organization, and knew not only who to involve in problem solving, but how to get those resources at the table. Her combination of quality know-how, operational expertise, and organizational savvy proved to be invaluable during the Orthopedic Center's transformation.

Once we knew we were beginning with Orthopedics (based upon both need and leadership), it was time to choose the physician whose practice would be the first to undergo the Lean transformation. Ultimately, we selected pediatric orthopedic surgeon Dr. Channing Tassone to be the Lean champion within the Orthopedic Center.

Dr. Tassone had a much different skill set. He was well-respected by his team and had fostered an atmosphere of open communication among the nurses, nurse practitioners, and other staff members who supported him. He was also open to trying new ideas and learning more about business leadership skills and quality improvement. He was an excellent public speaker who could help to spread the message of Lean within the organization. Finally and perhaps most importantly, he expressed a willingness to be part of the work—all of which pointed to him as a good choice for a Lean champion.

As he wryly explains: "I suspect I was probably seen as a willing victim, eager to try something different."

"Willing victims" like Dr. Tassone are important. Particularly in the initial stages of a Lean transformation, the one-doctor-at-a-time approach works precisely because the doctors pull it—it is not pushed upon them by a quality function or an executive. And so the physician who becomes the Lean champion must be willing to roll up her sleeves and dive into the work of the team, as Dr. Tassone says, "eager to try something different." The work cannot be delegated or ignored, or the rest of the practice's staff will take their cue from the doctor and no progress will be made.

If you are considering a physician who is reluctant to take the lead and be the champion, you probably should move on and find someone else. Do not spend energy trying to convince a physician who is unwilling. Instead, find a doctor who can be enthusiastic about the project and start there. The decision becomes a critical part of your strategy.

About the doctor as a Lean champion

So, why one doctor at a time? Why not just say "one manager at a time," or "one nurse"?

We approach Lean one *doctor* at a time because in the process of delivering care, the doctor is the critical element. The doctor essentially runs a mini-practice within a hospital setting or a medical group. How that doctor manages his practice has a tremendous impact on outcomes, efficiencies, patient satisfaction, patient access, and staff morale for the entire practicing group. While each physician practice is unique (even within the same clinic or hospital environment), Lean changes center around the doctor. That doctor must be part of, and function within, whatever changes are made. She cannot delegate the Lean project or opt out of participation.

Because it will change the very environment in which she is practicing, each doctor must consciously decide to go down the Lean path. Lean cannot be driven top down, nor can it go around the physician to focus on the rest of the staff. The physician's role is central, and the commitment and drive must come from the physician level.

Dr. Tassone believes that doctors leading the transformation have to be both committed and adaptable.

"Flexible—you have to be flexible," he tells other doctors considering Lean. "But at the same time, you also have to be a strong enough personality to say: 'Here are the things that need to keep happening.' And you also should be a person who's willing to stand up and say, 'This works.' You need to be someone who is willing to get out there and express how well it works."

Such doctor-to-doctor endorsement of the changes has much more credibility than someone outside the medical field (such as a consultant) saying, "This works." That, too, helps pull the initiative to other areas in a way that will increase its successes. The doctor is the leader of the practice; if she is on board and driving the changes, her actions send a powerful message about the importance of the improvement efforts. It is unfortunately very easy for organizational changes to be ignored or disparaged, but a respected leader who personally drives change can move mountains.

One of the many ways Dr. Tassone and Terry Schwartz (the program administrator) accomplished this was by together presenting programs about the benefits of Lean to the hospital's medical leadership group—though they wisely resisted making any of these presentations until they had hard data to share documenting the success.

And when Dr. Tassone talked informally with fellow doctors about the transformation, he says: "The biggest thing I found myself repeating was: 'Give it a try. Don't be scared off by the fact that they are going to ask you to do things differently than you have. All of us were skeptical at first.'"

SOME BACKGROUND: WHY PICK A STARTING POINT, OR MODEL LINE?

Lean initiatives often fail in the healthcare setting, in part due to the strategy used for their implementation. The favored approach is to start too big, either with broad training to which everyone is subjected or with projects in a dozen different areas. Once the training is completed (and forgotten) or the organization realizes it cannot manage a dozen projects, Lean becomes just another failed initiative and the staff says, "*I told you so.*"

Our alternative approach is to very precisely pick a starting point, or model line, and grow from there once some success has been achieved. "Model line" is a manufacturing term; it refers to one assembly line on which the Lean changes are trialed, so that the team implementing the changes can observe their efficacy and impact in a controlled setting. Those small changes are what builds the new system.

As the changes are trialed and then either adopted or abandoned on the model line, the model line begins to garner the attention of the rest of the organization because of the improvements it achieves. It becomes truly a model for other areas within the organization, attracting internal "tourists" who come to see it in operation and take what they've learned back to their areas to start their own work. The operators on that model line have opportunities to become spokespeople for Lean, describing how their processes have changed and what the impact of those changes has been.

In healthcare, because each physician practice is unique, the physician's practice becomes the model line. Starting with just one physician allows the Lean team to quickly and easily trial small changes, personalize them for the physician practice, and build an effective and successful Lean system. That system is customized for exactly what the physician needs and the circumstances of that practice, even while it shares characteristics with Lean systems in general, because it was created solely in the context of that practice with the direct involvement of the physician and his staff. That kind of change cannot be achieved through broad, multi-area rollouts or massive training efforts.

Note that the model line is not always the area that needs change the most. The model line serves several purposes. First, it is an opportunity to make significant improvements that affect patient outcomes, patient satisfaction, and staff satisfaction. Second, it is a "learning lab" where internal Lean expertise can be developed in a small area with a controlled scope. Finally, it's the test case to which everyone else looks to see whether Lean will "work" in the hospital or clinic. Those purposes cannot be achieved if the team is unwilling, or if the physician delegates involvement, or if the manager knows nothing of leading quality project teams—no matter how great the area's need for improvement. Start where you have not only the need, but also a capable manager and an enthusiastic physician.

Benefits (and limitations) of the approach

Working with just one model line—one doctor—inherently limits the scope of the Lean initiative. That's because the goal is not to blanket the organization with projects or training, but to delve the proverbial mile deep into one area. With that smaller scope, then, the Lean team can conduct quick trials of small changes and get immediate feedback about how those changes impact efficiency and patient care. Successful changes can be easily adapted by the team; unsuccessful ones have a limited impact and can be immediately abandoned. The smaller scope means that a smaller number of people will be involved with the Lean transformation. That small team can trial changes quickly, creating the Lean system in less time than an initiative involving many people could.

I will provide examples of our successful changes in Dr. Tassone's clinic as we expand upon the six success steps in the next section of this book, but there were also failed attempts. Fortunately, even this *ability to fail* highlights the benefits inherent in the one-doctor-at-a-time approach to Lean. Why? Because when someone on the team has an idea or hypothesis about how to improve efficiency, you can test it quickly, adapting it as needed.

In one case, no adaptation was needed because this particular idea failed so miserably. It went something like this: one of the scheduling difficulties Dr. Tassone and his team faced was being able to give new patients the time they needed during the busy clinic day. I suggested completely segregating the new patients, setting aside a period of several hours when Dr. Tassone would see only new patients.

Sadly, I did not know enough about the reality of how the clinic operated. I assumed most new patients would bring along x-rays and other diagnostic material, but the truth was that most did not. They would be sent off to radiology for x-rays, while Dr. Tassone…well, he didn't go in to a different exam room to see a follow-up patient who might have required only ten minutes of his time. None of those patients was scheduled during this period! Instead, he was left to stand around, waiting, until eventually we looked at each other and laughed. It quickly became clear that this scheduling template would not work in this clinic, so we decided to abandon the approach.

My point? The ability to quickly test a hypothesis is integral to Lean success, and the one-doctor-at-a-time approach is a fundamental part of making this happen. In this case, we learned a lot from our experiment and only impacted one four-hour clinic.

Starting with just one doctor also means that the hospital or clinic can start making changes right away, without having to coordinate with many functions or negotiate broad approval for what those changes are. A motivated manager and a committed physician can take steps together to make positive changes to the care delivery system right now—not a year from now after the board approves the plan.

Remember that if the changes occur too slowly, people in the organization will lose interest and Lean will become just another failed initiative that "didn't work around here." The immediacy of being able to test out potential changes has another huge benefit: sometimes the thought of working through the larger organization to get Lean moving is too daunting to even begin work. Starting small makes it do-able.

MOVING ON, SLOWLY AND DELIBERATELY, AS SUCCESS BUILDS

Approaching Lean one doctor at a time is a deliberate, strategic decision that will help you be successful with Lean in your healthcare organization. One warning: often the ideas of Lean catch fire in an organization, and then suddenly the push is on to train everyone, get the word out, and start lots of projects. This is a well-intentioned response, but one that rarely translates into sustainable success.

Instead, we advocate a much more measured approach that scales up over time as success is *demonstrated*, not just *promised*. Remember: find an area—a model line—that has a culture of quality improvement upon which to build, a capable manager overseeing operations, and a physician with the clear potential to be a champion for Lean. Use this area as a learning lab to conduct small, quick experiments with the Lean tools and techniques described in the rest of this book. Then build the Lean system, one step at a time, with those changes. As the Lean system grows, find ways to let your physician champion talk about the changes and the successes and pull other physicians into the discussion about Lean. Use what you have learned on the model line to help the next physician transform with Lean.

Dr. Tassone describes the approach and its impact best: "It took me being a guinea pig and my colleagues seeing, 'Hey, that works," before everyone started saying: 'OK. We'll do that.'"

Nurse Tracie Brasch agrees. "We were the guinea pig team," she says. "As things changed for us, that's when the other doctors took notice. And they started raising their hands to get involved."

ACTION STEPS

- Identify a manager within your organization who has experience with quality improvement efforts and project teams.

- Within that manager's area, identify physicians who are potential Lean champions, who are open to feedback and direction, who have the respect of their teams, and who are recognized as leaders in the organization.

- Work with the area manager to identify a physician with whom to initiate the Lean work

- Do not spend energy convincing a naysayer to participate as the model line; move on to another candidate to be the Lean champion.

2

Focus on Patient
Wait Times

In the introduction to this book, I talked about the critical decision to focus on wait times as the key metric in healthcare. It seems like an obvious choice now, but there were other options at the time. Healthcare is saddled with metrics and standards and regulations, and there is no shortage of data collection. Data is collected on everything from patient demographics to outcomes to efficiencies; quality departments seem bogged down with requests for reports analyzing the vast amounts of data collected and stored in the typical healthcare organization.

We could have chosen to focus on patient satisfaction surveys. Or staff turnover rates. Or, best of all in the healthcare setting, on the rate of medical errors. We could have even developed a spreadsheet with all of these factors, plugging the details into a program that would spit out a number letting us track our success.

But the truth is this: taken as a whole, those numbers are overwhelming. Some feel completely out of your control. Many of them aren't immediate, and some are not easy to understand.

Amidst all the mind-boggling information that is available in healthcare, wait times are refreshingly simple. After all, wait times are easy to understand, and there is no arguing with them. Anyone can walk out to the waiting room and see people waiting. Anyone can see that when the waiting room is full with patients, everything else also gets a little crazy.

It turns out that wait time is a powerful metric to indicate the overall health of the healthcare delivery system, and long wait times can reveal root causes of inefficiency—from haphazard communication to outdated departmental structures to staff role confusion. In addition, wait time has a real and tangible meaning—it's a number with a direct connection to the efficiency of the clinic or practice, and it's a measure that the staff can influence directly. It gives nurses and physicians and front desk staff alike an easy question to ask: *Why did clinic run 45 minutes over tonight?* Talking about this can uncover a chain of inefficiencies, handoffs, and errors that requires the project team to work together for a tangible goal.

Focusing on wait times also helps the team develop the mindset needed to continue evaluating processes throughout the Lean transformation. If you are to build a patient-centered healthcare system, focusing every staff member on the waiting patient is a powerful way to both ensure great patient service and create a sense of urgency for patient flow. Orthopedic nurse Tracie Brasch says, describing this new mindset, "Every day now, we evaluate our clinic. It's just natural. 'How do you think today went?' And that might get us started talking: 'Maybe we need to develop some hip dysplasia spots in the schedule. Maybe we need to do this.'"

She continues: "It's not an exercise we do to make knee-jerk changes. It's just a natural thing we do now, to constantly reevaluate how we do things and how we can make things run more smoothly."

Simply put: by focusing on wait times, you can provide a question that everyone can ask and help answer. Wait times provide a measure everyone can understand—and one everyone can impact. Wait times provide a framework to develop a Lean mindset, focused on evaluating and improving.

And they're a measure that's conveniently a safe distance away from the sanctity of the examination room, where we're leaving the actual interaction between doctor and patient completely untouched. Our goal in reducing wait times is simply to get the patient in to see the doctor as quickly as possible—not in any way to impact or affect what happens from there.

Notes Dr. Tassone: "In my case, I wasn't worried about this impacting the quality of my patient care because I simply knew that I would not allow that to happen. Patient care—that depends upon me, that's all about how I provide it, and I knew I would never change that.

"But the thing that was so smart about all of this was that it never had anything to do with decreasing or changing patient care. We were looking for ways to add more value-added time between the patients and the physician. We were never going to attempt to be with patients less. It was simply about how I handled my time."

A waiting patient, whether for test results or antibiotics administration, also serves as a powerful motivator to transform the organization and create safer processes in the emergency departments, intensive care units, operating rooms, and support departments such as radiology, labs, echo, and others.

Using wait times as the key metric in your Lean transformation will help to ensure that the emphasis stays on straightforward, observable efficiency gains, regardless of the area or specialty or organization.

And, as an added benefit, it will provide a simple source of happiness for all of the workers: the ability to usually leave work on time. "It made them happier; it made their families happier," notes Dr. Tassone's administrative assistant, Amy Ricely.

WHY PATIENTS CARE ABOUT WAIT TIMES...AND WHY THEY DON'T

Lean changes seem enormous at the outset and present a daunting challenge; but wait times are a flag, a guidepost, a highly visible indicator of our performance. No other metric tells us the state of our processes so clearly.

However, I'd be misleading you if I didn't note that the dynamic between wait times and patient satisfaction is a complicated one. Yes, wait times are our integral measure for the healthcare staff undergoing a Lean transformation. But they're not necessarily the most important consideration to the patient. Because the truth is that patients are willing to wait—and still tend to leave satisfied—if they ultimately get quality time with their doctor. Patients don't necessarily mind waiting. Or at least they're certainly used to it!

To show you what I mean, I want to describe a training course we conducted with a healthcare client in 2009. We asked the participants to be "patients" in simulated clinic visits. We took them to an actual clinic, assigned them an ailment, and let them experience the process from the patient's point of view. Some sat at check-in for ten or 15 minutes. Others waited in exam rooms just as long or longer. We made them wait again if they needed care from multiple providers, like an x-ray or tests. Eventually, though, they all saw the "physician" and the simulation ended.

Back in the classroom, we discussed their experiences and took a look at their visit times and wait times. "Patients" who spent an hour or more in the clinic saw the "physician" for an average of three minutes, while their wait times averaged 55 minutes. This was by design—the client organization had similar wait times and physician consultation times. Yet, the group's overwhelming response was that the wait times were acceptable. One participant—herself a healthcare professional—said, "The wait time was OK. I mean, I knew why I was waiting." Another called her 61-minute clinic visit and 3-minute physician consultation, "Not bad." A third said she enjoyed having time to read a magazine.

It's a dynamic healthcare professionals see all the time. As Dr. Tassone describes it: "Patients may say they don't like waiting at their doctor's office. But let them come into an empty waiting room and walk right in to see the doctor at their scheduled time, and I guarantee you they'll wonder about that doctor! Having to wait almost reassures them that they're seeing a 'good' doctor."

What does this mean? Why are patients apparently so willing to wait?

In their study, *"Willing to Wait? The influence of patient wait time on satisfaction,"* researchers Roger T. Anderson, Fabian T. Camacho, and Rajesh Balkrishnan conclude that long wait times, combined with short visit times with the doctor, resulted in the lowest overall patient satisfaction. The authors note, "Our study suggests that long waiting times and short visit times are a toxic combination for patient satisfaction and one that providers and practice managers should avoid if they are concerned about patient-centered measures of healthcare quality such as patient satisfaction."

Clearly the ability to reduce wait times without rushing the physician from patient to patient is the Holy Grail of patient satisfaction. It appears that patients are willing to wait—or at least accustomed to waiting—so long as they ultimately get quality time with their doctor.

Does that mean we should back off from our focus on wait times? I'd argue the opposite. It seems to me that this mindset instead is both the reason for and the challenge of attacking wait times in healthcare processes. We have grown accustomed to waiting when we visit healthcare providers, so much so that even long waits seem normal and acceptable. In fact, our simulated patients got upset about wait times only if someone who came into the clinic after them got called to see the doctor before they did.

This complacency about wait times has dramatic implications for healthcare when you consider that similar complacency and low expectations have caused the demise of other industries!

In order to successfully transform our healthcare processes with Lean, we need to generate a sense of urgency each day in the physician practice. Lean is about the relentless pursuit of perfection—that is the feeling we need to bring to Lean efforts in healthcare. It is not OK to expect patients to wait. It is not acceptable to lower our expectations about the service we provide.

And there's another compelling reason to focus on wait times as we undergo Lean transformations. In the study cited just previously, the authors describe the physician's available time as a fixed asset, meaning that the more time the physician spends with any individual patient, the longer other patients will have to wait.

I'm going to challenge that premise in the very next chapter, when I discuss our first success step, creating physician flow. I maintain that when focusing on wait times as the metric and using Lean principles to reduce wait time, the physician's time is no longer a fixed asset. Lean can actually create time during the day, so that the wait times are reduced even as time available for patient consultations increases.

In other words, wait times are reduced when the many and varied sources of waste are removed from the care delivery process. And when the waste is removed from the work of the physician and staff, everyone has more time to focus on what matters: quality patient care.

"Since the changes, it feels like I can take that extra time to help that crying mom or patient," explains Lori Seubert, the orthopedic nurse. "Everything continues, versus everything stopping in the past until you're done with the extra minutes in that room with your patients.

"Our patients feel taken care of, and that's huge for all of us," she says. "All of us are not in it for any other reason."

Remember, this ability to focus on patient care is the true goal of efforts to improve efficiency. And it's one all healthcare professionals find valuable.

Some background about Children's Hospital of Wisconsin and its Orthopedic Center:

Children's Hospital of Wisconsin, founded in 1894, is recognized as one of the leading pediatric healthcare centers in the United States. It is rated No. 3 in the nation by *Parents* magazine and named one of America's Best Children's Hospitals by *U.S. News & World Report.* Children's Hospital of Wisconsin is a Level I Pediatric Trauma Center verified by the American College of Surgeons. The hospital has been redesignated a Magnet hospital by the American Nurses Credentialing Center, a national honor that recognizes nursing excellence. Private, independent, and not-for-profit, the hospital serves children and families from Wisconsin, the Upper Peninsula of Michigan, northern Illinois, and beyond. Children's Hospital is the flagship member of Children's Hospital and Health System.

Children's Hospital and Health System is an independent healthcare system dedicated solely to the health and well-being of children. For more information, visit the Web site at www.chw.org.

About the Orthopedic Center (Outcomes Report):
Compared with other hospitals in the Pediatric Health Information System, the Orthopedic Center at Children's Hospital of Wisconsin:

• Has consistently maintained a higher volume of spinal fusion patients compared to the average of PHIS peers in the last several years

• Performs more than twice as many pediatric spinal fusions than any other group of orthopedic surgeons in Wisconsin

• Charges significantly less for orthopedic inpatient stays and spinal fusions than the average of PHIS peers

• Has a significantly lower average severity-adjusted charge per visit for all orthopedic patients and spinal fusion patients than the average of PHIS peers

• Has one of the only electromagnetic pediatric gait labs to be used clinically in the region

WAIT TIMES ARE THE STARTING POINT, BUT HOW DO YOU BEGIN?

Focusing on wait times is how you get started on a Lean transformation. At the outset, a Lean transformation can seem overwhelming and difficult to set into motion. Much of the literature about Lean transformation focuses on settings where the changes have already taken place. Those stories can be inspirational, but they sometimes lack the concrete advice you need to replicate that success. The focus on wait times is a solid, meaningful, and important place to start; it is how you diagnose your processes to find the root causes of inefficiency and begin to make meaningful change.

To begin:

• Collect data about one physician practice.

• Conduct a waste walk in that practice's physical space.

• Create a value stream map.

COLLECT DATA ABOUT ONE PHYSICIAN PRACTICE

The first step in changing the paradigm about wait times is to collect data to highlight the problem. It is easy to ignore the current state, or assume that the problem is everyone else's and not yours, when there is no specific data about your process.

In Chapter One, we talked about finding a physician champion to begin the Lean transformation. This step of data collection is an excellent way to engage that physician because it helps to diagnose the specific issues that physician practice is facing. Notes Orthopedic program administrator Terry Schwartz: "This is an eye-opening moment for a doctor—to see that someone may have spent 60 minutes at your clinic but only received two or three minutes of your time. It's really something that gets their attention."

This step is so important because each practice is unique, just as each physician is unique. A doctor's personality and interpersonal style influences the practice's work environment; his personal preferences dictate a lot about the work methods. The practice is further defined by the demographics and conditions of the patients the physician sees. Even the physical set up of the practice space plays a role in differentiating one physician practice from another. The reality is that data from someone else's practice (or worse, generalized data) will not be compelling to your physician champion.

In other words, the data must be specific to the individual physician, just as the resulting solutions must be customized to the particular practice. So begin with individual diagnosis.

To do this, set aside a four-hour block of time and collect data through direct observation of the practice. Our goal is to collect a statistically significant set of data, typically 15–30 patients. Using a watch and a pencil, take note of each patient who comes into the waiting room and the time that patient spends at each step of the process. How long does each patient spend at check-in? In the waiting room? In the exam room? With follow-up care providers? How long does the patient visit with the physician? Collecting these times for a four-hour window should provide an accurate snapshot of the process's current state. When that data, collected through pencil-and-paper observation, is presented to the physician or care team, a powerful case for change is built.

This data can also be powerful for the physician champion. If, for example, that physician saw 40 patients in the four-hour observation window—each for an average of three minutes—that leaves two hours of the physician's time unaccounted for. Although the physician may have been busy during that time, from the patient point of view, nothing productive happened. That kind of data often convinces the physician that there is indeed time during the day that could be better spent, and that there is opportunity for improvement.

Conduct a waste walk to look for underlying causes

The waste walk is the next step in the process; it begins the search for underlying causes of long wait times and other frustrations in the system. In a waste walk, the Lean team physically walks through the practice area with the goal of identifying sources of waste in the care delivery system.

Lean defines waste as anything that takes up resources but provides no value. There are many good books available about Lean basics, including the definitions of the different categories of waste (we recommend *Lean Thinking* by James Womack and Daniel Jones). For our purposes, we will define them quickly:

- **Motion:** people having to move excessively to do their jobs, such as walking too far for a piece of equipment or to collect necessary tools, or wasting time because workstations are not laid out with the job in mind.

- **Waiting:** wasted time in which a worker (physician, nurse, assistant, and so on) has to wait to complete a step because information, space, or authority are missing.

- **Over Processing:** wasted steps in the process—steps that may be redundant or done simply because they always have been; for example, transcribing what someone else has written.

- **Defects:** mistakes that take time and resources to be corrected, or that cause the product to be discarded.

- **Transportation:** wasted movement of equipment, often because of where or how the equipment is stored.

- **Inventory:** having so much equipment and supplies that it becomes difficult to store and manage, or not having the right items on hand when they are needed (often these two circumstances happen at the same time).

- **Overproduction:** making or processing more of something than the next step in the process can handle, thus causing those things (or people) to wait in between steps.

Table 2.1 is a sample waste walk form. The team conducting the waste walk uses this form as an observation worksheet to capture as many examples of waste in the physician practice as they can. When I conduct waste walks at the beginning of Lean work in an area, I always get the same reaction from the project team. Initially, they are skeptical of the process. At the end, they are surprised by just how much waste they find. I routinely hear comments such as, "I never realized how far we had to walk for supplies!" or "We make patients walk to too many different areas!"

For example, you might discover that paperwork is being filled out but never used. You might discover the need to clarify x-ray orders—especially if different physicians have different preferences on how these are completed. You might find that the Physician's Assistant is simply catching the doctor between exam rooms for clarifications, when what's really needed is a planned handoff. You may find wasted steps because supplies run out more quickly than expected. There may be a simple lack of communication between the clinic assistants and others, resulting in long wait times in exam rooms. In short, the project team opens its eyes to the waste all around them and the need for improvement, and a very valuable opportunity for change is created.

One of the main reasons waste walks are so effective in healthcare is that healthcare professionals are clinicians, not Lean engineers. They are not specifically trained to think of their processes in terms of steps and flow, waste and value. When I began my career as a young process engineer, the valve or the pump or the project I was working on became my sole focus—I never thought about how that piece fit into the larger process of providing value to a customer. Seeing the entire value stream, rather than one isolated part, is a learned skill—one that the simple waste walk is very effective at teaching.

Or, as Pediatric Intensive Care physician Dr. Theresa Mikhailov, who helped with our Lean transformation underway in the PICU, explains: "You have no idea how much waste there is in healthcare until you take a waste walk through your own unit. Wasted motion, wasted time, wasted inventory—it's all there."

Table 2.1 Sample waste walk form.

7 Wastes	Why is it there? Possible solution?
Motion: Staff looking for information, other staff members, materials, supplies, forms, and so on to service the patients or complete tasks.	
Waiting: Staff waiting for patients, procedures, each other, surgeries, reports, and equipment, to finish the next step in their job.	
Over Processing: Redundant checks, questions, clarifications, duplicate paperwork, inconsistent procedures, excessive tests, and so on.	
Defects: Poorly scheduled patients, patient service failures, paperwork errors, medication errors, incorrect billing / charges, preventable mistakes, and so on.	
Transportation: Unnecessary movement of patients, equipment, supplies, materials, information, and so on.	
Inventory: Stuffing of medications and supplies, missing supplies, uncontrolled inventories in stock rooms or warehouses, poor replenishment systems, missing forms, and so on.	
Overproduction: Working on patients, information, and procedures significantly before the next process or person is ready.	

Waste walks have the added benefit of easily involving everyone in the practice in root cause analysis. Involving the team early and often will help to avoid the finger-pointing and resistance that the staff will naturally feel when someone else tries to "correct" their jobs.

"It doesn't seem possible at first," notes Dr. Tassone, "but suddenly you are enlightened to things you never would have perceived.

VALUE STREAM MAPPING PROVIDES THE OVERVIEW

The next step in the process is value stream mapping. The value stream map is a 40,000-foot view of the steps and processes required to fulfill patient needs. (See Figure 2.1.) It is like taking the roof off of the building and looking down to identify where we interact with the patient and where the patient waits for the next step to occur. Without value stream mapping, changes can be disjointed, suboptimized, and ultimately ineffectual. A value stream map illustrates how each change affects the overall system and builds towards achieving the future state. This tool can make the difference between a real and meaningful Lean transformation and inconsequential (but nonetheless expensive) Lean activity.

It's a difference I've seen again and again in manufacturing. I visited one manufacturer in the aerospace industry that undertook a great deal of Lean activity but neglected to complete a value stream map to tie all of that activity together and envision their future, ideal process. As a result, one tool—5S—took over. They created taped lines on the floor to show workers where to store the inventory that resulted from their unbalanced schedules and they had shiny piles of unwanted product in the warehouse, but fundamentally, nothing about their process had changed.

I have often heard it said that Lean principles do not apply in healthcare, or that only superficial changes in healthcare settings can be made with Lean tools. I've found that those comments come mostly from healthcare organizations that attempted a Lean transformation without a future state value stream map. Where physicians and their teams have taken the time to map out what their processes could look like without all the waste and confusion, the results are extraordinary. The map gives them a powerful communication tool to share the vision with the team and sponsors, and helps to sequence the implementation of tools. No other step in the launch of a Lean initiative is as critical. Don't skip it!

"When we started out this process of mapping…it suddenly became clear," notes Orthopedic nurse Tracie Brasch. "We started watching what we did: 'Now I have to go all the way back here for tape, and now there's no suture remover, and now I have to go all the way to the cast room, and now to x-ray…' To see this on paper, I guess my reaction was just: Wow.

And that's when it really hit me: this might make a difference. These are things we can do."

There are many resources available for learning to use value stream mapping. (*Learning To See,* by Mike Rother and Dan Shook, is a great introduction.) Essentially, there are two kinds of value stream maps: current state maps and future state maps. Both capture the patient flow as well as the information flow through the care process. They highlight where the patients stop flowing, resulting in wait times. They also capture critical metrics about the cycle time for each step in the process, where defects occur, and how much time in the process is value added compared to the overall lead time. The current state map is drawn using direct observation of the process as it operates today. The future state map is created by the Lean team as it envisions how the process could operate if the sources of waste were eliminated.

The future state map guides the work of the Lean team. The data collection, waste walks, and current state value stream mapping all help the team understand what impedes flow and causes patients to wait. Armed with that understanding, the team then redraws the map to eliminate those impediments and achieve flow, thereby reducing patient wait times. We have laid out the six success steps specifically to help you envision that future state for your process. Each success step introduces a tool or concept of Lean—in a sequence proven effective for healthcare—that will eliminate the common flow impediments you will find on your current state map.

We have made one critical adaptation to value stream mapping for healthcare. In order to provide a useful lead time metric to hospitals and clinics, we have defined lead time as the total amount of time the patient spends in a healthcare facility. The value-added time is the amount of time spent with the physician and any follow-up service providers. Therefore, the clinic patient who spends 50 minutes in the clinic, sees the physician for a total of five minutes, and spends five minutes getting a cast on has a value-added percentage of 20 percent. We have defined value-added time in this limited way based on our knowledge that shorter wait times and more time with the providers contribute to higher patient satisfaction.

Focusing on wait time shifts focus back to the patient

To summarize: patient wait times are the most valuable metric in your Lean efforts. Focusing on wait times helps to change the point of view from the provider to the healthcare consumer—the ultimate customer. Without that focus, we too easily accept the current state of our processes and lose the sense of urgency about improvements that drives the greatest transformations. So be the patient for a while and see the process through those eyes. Doing so will build the case for change and help you begin your successful Lean journey.

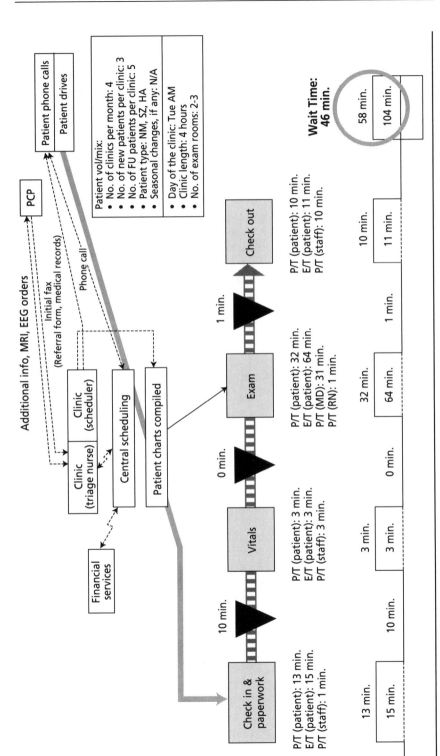

Figure 2.1 Value stream map.

As you continue your Lean transformation, you might want to consider the long-term benefits of Lean, as outlined by Children's corporate vice president Larry Duncan.

"Lean gives your staff a greater feeling of community. You have common goals. You're given tools that work to make things happen, to see improvement," Duncan says. "Lean has really evened the playing field, because everyone has received the same training, they're all speaking the same language. It's not driven from the top down. It's about a work community coming together to make changes that actually make things better."

ACTION STEPS

- Collect wait time data from the physician champion's practice.

- Conduct a waste walk through the practice area.

- Create a current state value stream map and begin to envision the future state.

The Six Success Steps

3

Step 1 – Create Physician Flow

So you've chosen your Lean physician champion—whether in one area or multiple areas. You've taken steps to document the processes there as they are now, and to envision how things could look in the future. Now it's time to begin making some changes. Our first Success Step is to create physician flow. This simply means to create processes that allow the doctor to move from one patient to the next in an efficient manner, with the correct information in hand and clear direction.

At this point, you might expect me to talk a bit about the backlog at Dr. Tassone's clinic, or how harried his staff were, or even how they tracked the progress of patients from his office to x-ray and back again. Instead, I'm going to begin with a story that seemingly has nothing to do with Children's Hospital, or Dr. Tassone's Orthopedic Center, or the Lean transformation we undertook there. (But don't worry: It's in keeping with our focus on a value stream approach, on seeing and reviewing processes from the patient point of view.)

Several years ago, I made an appointment to see a primary care physician because I thought I had pneumonia. I was new in the area and did not know the doctor well. Once at the office, I waited long past my appointment time, but since it was the flu season and the office was busy, I did not think that the wait was exceptional. (Sound familiar?) Once I was in an exam room, I explained my symptoms and history of pneumonia—which I had been diagnosed with three or four times in the past five years—to the person who came to take my vitals. I explained this again to the nurse who came in while I was waiting for the doctor.

The doctor came into the exam room 45 minutes after my scheduled appointment. She seemed to consult some notes. She examined me. When I mentioned toward the end of our consultation how many times I had had pneumonia, she couldn't hide her irritation. *"When were you going to tell me that?"* she asked. I can imagine she left the exam room feeling frustrated at patients who don't give her the information she needs for a solid diagnosis. I know I left annoyed and wary, uncertain that I had received the best possible care.

Of course, almost everyone who has ever been to a doctor has a story like this, about those long wait times and about critical information that did not get passed along, about busy doctors' offices and the feeling of being shuffled around, about the worry that something got missed in the process. These stories undermine confidence in the care process and erode patient satisfaction.

Julie Pedretti, Children's Hospital's director of public relations and marketing, explains this dynamic: "When patient families have really good experiences, they do talk about that with other families, with their friends, with their neighbors, their relatives," she notes. "When they have experiences that are not so positive, when they've waited for 15 minutes, 40 minutes, or one-and-a-half hours for care and they feel like they haven't been communicated with, that is the kind of experience that they also talk about in the community and that's not a good thing."

She adds: "Those perceptions stay on for very long time. It costs the organization a lot of money to change those perceptions—to let families know, to let the referring physicians know, that the services today are what they would expect them to be."

And so this patient-focused perspective is important—in fact, it is vital—at this stage of the Lean transformation process because our goal here, as we take our initial steps to create physician flow, is to see the process from the patient's point of view. It's essential for everyone undergoing a Lean transformation in healthcare to understand what is important to patients evaluating the quality of the care they were given, and ultimately to focus on providing that value-added service without waste.

> "Word of mouth is the main way the reputation of a hospital is communicated. Patients are likely to first seek the advice of friends and family members when selecting a healthcare provider. ... Hospitals that are highly recommended by patients as a good place to receive care are typically also lauded by their employees and physicians."
>
> From the 2007 *Hospital Check-Up Report—Physician Perspectives on American Hospitals*, published by Press Ganey Associates, Inc, 2007

Here, again, we start with the physician because the physician has to make the ultimate decision regarding the patient diagnosis. Quite simply: The patient is in the clinic to see the doctor. In a clinic setting, where there are always multiple patients for a physician, the physician also becomes the driver of the patient care process. And as you know, a quality interaction with the physician is one of the primary determiners of patient satisfaction.

(As we've discussed, research tells us that the time with the doctor in the exam room is the most important value-added portion of the clinic visit. That study we cited earlier, published in 2007 by BMC Health Services Research, showed that time spent with the physician was the strongest predictor of patient satisfaction. Although longer wait times were associated with lower satisfaction, as you'll recall it was the combination of long waiting time with a short doctor visit that was associated with very low patient satisfaction.)

Given that quality time with the physician is the part that patients value most, it would be logical for healthcare organizations to make sure each physician has enough time to meet those expectations. However, many organizations reward physicians based on number of patients seen or revenue generated, which would seem to decrease the time available for each doctor-patient interaction. Also, some clinics and practices are simply busy, sometimes to an overwhelming degree. The physician is responsible for file dictations and other paperwork that further cut into the available time. Because physician days are already long, it is clear that making more time available for patient interactions will require fundamentally changing the way the clinic operates.

ANALYZE HOW THE PHYSICIAN WORKS AS PART OF LARGER PROCESS

At Children's Hospital during our Lean transformation process, Terry Schwartz, the Orthopedic program administrator, noted that the most eye-opening moment for many physicians reluctant to undertake the process came when she tracked and then shared with them the amount of time patients spent at the clinic (often up to an hour) compared with the amount of time spent consulting with the doctor (often as little as three minutes).

These numbers are not at all unusual in a busy Orthopedic Center that is often running behind schedule or chronically overbooked. Patients will have to wait to be roomed, wait to have a cast removed and x-rays taken, and wait again to see the doctor. And although Dr. Tassone noted that he'll give his patients the exact same quality of care during the time he spends in an exam room with them, improving the process—or adding value—clearly benefits everyone.

In Lean parlance, the total amount of time spent in the clinic is called lead time. When the value-added time (time spent with the physician) is divided by the lead time (overall time the patient spends in the clinic) the resulting metric paints a picture of what portion of time is spent in value-added activities. In the case of our busy fractures clinic—with a lead time of 60 minutes, an average physician consultation time of three minutes, and casting or other services time of let's say six minutes—we find that the value-added time for the patient is only 15 percent of the visit. This is not an unusual result; no matter what the industry, we find that no more than five to 15 percent of time spent in a given process is value added. And we find that often the value-added time is significantly less.

At the beginning of the Lean transformation, we need to analyze how the physician operates as part of the larger process of providing patient care. This analysis sometimes strikes our clients as an uncomfortable one: After all, physicians are highly educated and practicing what can be viewed as an art as much as a science. However, remember that our analysis focuses not on the consultation between patient and physician in the exam room, but on everything that happens during the entire visit.

When we focus on the process of getting the physician into the exam room with all the necessary information and without wasted time, everyone wins. The doctor's job becomes easier because problems and hassles are taken out of her way. The clinic staff members reduce "fire fighting" and frustration and stay on schedule. And most importantly, the patient gets the care he needs without unnecessary delays or confusion.

"As the primary source of all patient referrals and as leaders of the healthcare team, physicians play a vital role in the hospital's overall performance. Hospitals that effectively build solid relationships with their physicians benefit from a consistent patient flow. Due to high physician demand, unsatisfied physicians can be easily drawn to a competing facility. Hospitals that successfully meet the needs of their physicians enjoy both financial and clinical benefits.

"The National Physician Priority Index identifies what doctors say hospital administrators can do to better meet the expectations of physicians. The number one priority for improvement is how the administration responds to the needs and ideas of physicians."

From the *2007 Hospital Check-Up Report—Physician Perspectives on American Hospitals*, published by Press Ganey Associates, Inc, 2007.

CREATING FLOW FOR THE PHYSICIAN

So, because of that direct link between shorter wait times, quality physician-patient interactions, and patient satisfaction, our Lean transformation starts with the physician. The physician is the centerpiece of the process, and the goal is to make the physician *flow* from one patient to another.

Flow is a Lean term that describes an ideal state in which the thing going through a process—whether that thing is a product or a part, a service or even a person—never stops moving from beginning to end.

Flow is easy to visualize in manufacturing. Flow in automotive manufacturing means that the conveyor belt does not stop moving at any point in assembly of the vehicle until that car is delivered to the waiting customer. Compare that image to the reality of manufacturing in which flow is interrupted by problems, defects, or distance, resulting in parts and subassemblies that are stacked up and stored in aisles and warehouses, and in which even finished cars and trucks are stored on huge lots waiting to be sold. The wastes in that process are enormous and costly—all those parts and subassemblies and finished goods have to be moved around and managed and can be lost or damaged in the process. Worst of all, customer requirements can change in the time it takes that vehicle to get to the sales floor, making the entire process a wasteful exercise.

In healthcare, we find a similar scenario. Flow means that a patient comes into the clinic, is immediately checked in and roomed, has any diagnostic tests or x-rays performed, is seen by the physician, receives a diagnosis and care plan, and leaves. The reality in healthcare is not that simple, however, and many factors interrupt flow. In the clinic environment, flow can be interrupted by patients who are scheduled in the wrong clinic or for the wrong amount of time, by emergencies that are squeezed onto an already full schedule, or by administrative tasks that the clinic team is expected to fit in between patients. Flow also can be interrupted by the doctor not having the information she needs when entering a patient's room, or by not having a clear sense of which patient is ready to be seen next.

When the goal is to create physician flow, we apply the same concept of flow in the Lean manufacturing sense to the physician's work. The ideal is to have the physician move from one patient to the next with the right information in hand and in a calm, controlled environment. We look for all of the issues that stop the physician and result in patients that queue up in the waiting room or at supplying processes such as radiology. These issues are many, since clinic processes are rarely set up with physician flow in mind. For reasons ranging from regulation to internal policies, clinic processes contain too many handoffs, role confusion among clinic staff, physical separation of departments, and informal (and therefore unreliable) communications—all of which results in the physician walking into an exam room behind schedule and without the information she needs to conduct a quality consultation with the patient.

So, how do we begin? First we have to step into our steel-toed boots and borrow some concepts that originated in manufacturing: shared resources and changeover. Then we have to create a tool called a Lean process map.

SHARED RESOURCES
(HOW THE PHYSICIAN'S TIME IS SCHEDULED)

A shared resource is typically one specialized machine through which products from many different lines must flow. For example, an automotive plant that sends all painted parts through a central oven would consider that oven a shared resource. Shared resources are potential pacemakers in the process; if that shared resource is behind schedule or unavailable, everything else waits.

In the clinic, the physician sees all types of patients in a given clinic type. There is typically one doctor in the clinic, not one for each exam room. Because all patients must flow "through" the physician, we treat the physician as a shared resource. That means paying special attention to how the physician's time is scheduled.

The schedule of products going to that shared resource must be level; one product cannot monopolize its time and make all others wait. That automotive plant would not (or at least should not) cure only rear-view mirrors in its oven and let the painted doors and fenders stack up. Nor can the physician see back-to-back new or complex cases while quick follow-up appointments are made to wait. Scheduling templates often reflect the personal preferences of the physician; clinic end times are a good way to verify that a provider's scheduling template is working effectively. If the clinic consistently ends late, the template should be adjusted to ensure that the physician can work effectively with the interval between appointments and the mix of patient types.

Although the scheduling template dictates in what interval the patients arrive at the clinic, the concept of a FIFO lane determines in what order the patients are seen in the exam rooms. (See Figure 3.1.) FIFO stands for "First In First Out." It's a concept frequently used to schedule shared resources in manufacturing. Products that must flow through a shared resource queue up in a FIFO lane and are processed in that order, rather than by some other priority (or randomly).

In the clinic, a FIFO lane mentality dictates that the next patient who is ready in the exam room is clearly identified for the physician. Ideally, the "next ready patient" is the one the physician sees next. A FIFO lane means there is a clear system in place to identify the next ready patient so that the physician does not need to decide whom to see next, nor does she choose an exam room to enter at random. Remember we talked about saving a minute here and a minute there in the introduction; valuable time is lost for the physician in the process of deciding which patient to see next, gathering that patient's paperwork, and actually walking into an exam room. Because patient arrival times and needs can vary greatly, appointment times do not always indicate the next ready patient. A FIFO lane is a more reliable system. Leveling the schedule and seeing patients on a first in/first out basis will help ensure that the most valuable resource (the shared resource) is able to utilize his or her time most efficiently while in the clinic.

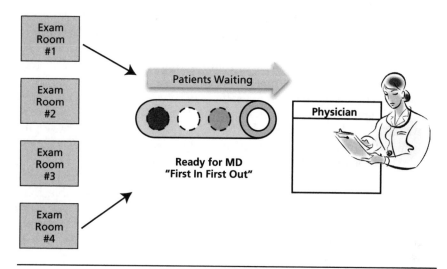

Figure 3.1 FIFO lane illustration.

CHANGEOVER

In manufacturing, the operator usually works at a machine to perform his part of the process. A physician consulting with a patient can be seen as both the operator and the machine. In fact, the physician is not just a machine in our analogy: he or she is the only machine through which all of the product must flow.

A manufacturing firm that had only one machine would take great care to ensure that all of its available time was used to process product. One of the ways that manufacturing companies do this is to focus on the changeover of the machine between parts. Changeover refers to the time it takes to finish one task and get ready to begin the next. In our automotive plant, changeover refers to elapsed time between producing the last driver's side rear-view mirror and retooling the machines to produce the first passenger side rear-view mirror. In the airline industry, changeover refers to the time it takes to unload passengers, clean the cabin of the aircraft, refuel, restock, and load baggage in preparation for the next group of passengers.

In the clinic, there is changeover between patients for the physician. Changeover begins when the physician finishes one patient's consultation. Changeover ends when the physician walks into the exam room to see the next patient. While the physician is with the first patient, the next patient must be prepared for the physician's consultation. He or she must be ready in an exam room, complete with paperwork, radiology films, and all necessary information. Viewed this way, most of the activity of the non-provider staff can be seen as changeover.

Changeover time is called "internal" if it happens while the machine is stopped. Internal changeover causes delays in the system because the machine is not running and the product has stopped flowing. The goal is to move the changeover tasks from internal to external, so that they happen in parallel and the machine is idle for as little time as possible. A racing pit crew is a great visual example of internal changeover. In order to keep the racecar off the track for only seconds, rather than minutes, the crew has everything ready before the driver makes the pit stop. When the driver pulls in, all of the equipment needed for the changeover is right where it is needed, and the crew is focused on a single goal.

In the clinic, the goal is to make as much of the changeover external as possible. This means taking a critical look at all of the tasks that must be accomplished in the process of patient care, both before and after the physician consultation, and performing them in parallel. While the physician is with one patient, the next patient should be prepped and all necessary information gathered. In addition to the patient preparation, a timely and standard handoff is an important part of the changeover process. A focus on changeover can result in time savings of minutes per patient; multiplying those minutes by 40 patients a day can mean hours in terms of clinic end times.

It is important to note that the reduced wait times and other time savings do not come from shorter patient-doctor visits or from imposing target consultation times on the physicians. When we view the physician as an operator of a machine performing a value-added process, Lean tells us to look at changeovers and non-value-added times instead of at the physician-patient interaction. When we reduce this non-patient facing physician time in a clinic to a minimum, not only does the clinic begin to end on time, it also opens up opportunities for the physician to increase patient volumes or create emergent slots or increase patient-physician consultation times to form deeper doctor-patient relationships— depending on the particular situation.

LEAN PROCESS MAPPING

Putting the concepts of shared resources and changeovers into action takes a bit of analysis and planning. We must take a closer look at the current process in which the physician is operating in order to find sources of waste. The value stream map described in the previous chapter gives us a high-level view of the entire process of providing patient care; however, the value stream map does not give us details about each step.

To come in for a closer view, we create a Lean process map. (See Figure 3.2.) This is a slightly modified version of the value stream map that focuses on individual staff members' workflow or other processes. The goal is to use value stream maps for all patient mapping and use

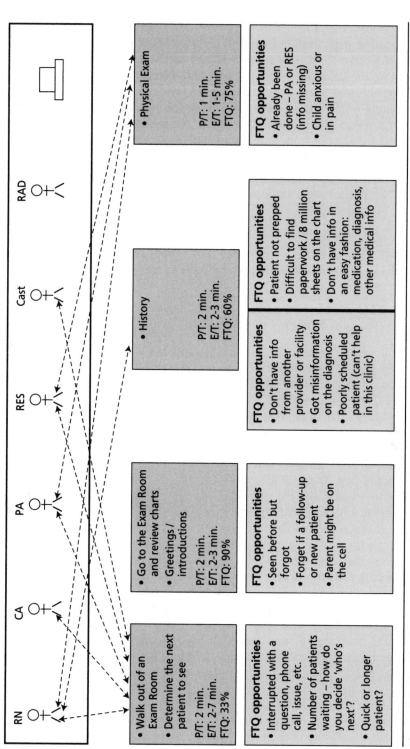

Figure 3.2 Physician lean process map (one patient flow).

Lean process maps for everything else. The Lean process map shows us the detailed steps of the process, as well as critical metrics about the time each step takes and how often that step is done right the first time. In addition, the Lean process map provides a picture of the communication among different roles in the clinic at each step.

Like a value stream map, a Lean process map can only be created through direct observation. Define the beginning and ending points of the process in question, and then observe it in action and capture the following information:

- Main steps of a staff member's workflow (in this case the detailed physician steps involved in going from patient to patient)

- P/T: Process time for each step (actual touch time for a particular task or face time with the patient)

- E/T: Elapsed time for each step (how long did the step actually take; this may mean searching for a nurse or information or the patient, for example)

- FTQ: First time quality (written as the percentage of time that the step goes right the first time)

Once the basic process information is captured, add the communication or information exchange that occurs for each step. From whom must the physician get information in order to advance to the next step in the process? For example, perhaps a nurse has the patient history, or the radiology tech has needed films. Or the physician needs information from the computer before he can proceed.

Finally, capture the reasons for any FTQ metric of less than 100 percent. The team will need to use its expertise to estimate how often that particular step does not happen as expected. For example, as he walks out of an exam room the physician needs a nurse to give the patient an excuse for school. Only 50 percent (or FTQ = 50 percent) of the time, the nurse is actually available outside the exam room. The other times she is busy with another patient or doing other tasks. As a result, you may decide in the short term to include a blank excuse form with the patient paperwork that the doctor has with him. For a long-term fix, you may want the nurse to overlap her time with the doctor toward the end of each patient's visit to ensure quick and efficient follow up for excuse, education, or other needs.

FTQ measures of less than 100 percent are evidence of the seven wastes in the process and provide a strong starting place for problem solving and change. Summarize the reasons on the map.

The Lean process map has the added benefit of being able to communicate problems with the current system with visual impact. Creating the map with the team responsible for making changes helps to dramatically increase understanding of the current state and commitment to the change process.

Although Lean process mapping is a diagnostic step aimed at helping you understand the current state of your operations, it often reveals immediate opportunities for change. These small (and often not so small) changes can motivate the team and help gain momentum for your improvement effort.

For example, a Lean process map we created with a client revealed a missing communication step after the physician was through seeing a patient. If the physician simply went on to the next exam room, no one knew whether the first patient was finished and could simply leave— especially if the nurse was not required for a follow-up discussion. The patients in these scenarios would stay in the exam room, expecting someone to tell them they could go, or would step out after a while to ask someone to check their status. It turns out that the patient could have left long ago, had the physician communicated that to the patient or to the staff. This missing step was obvious on the map, and led the team to create a whiteboard for communicating patient status. (We'll examine that idea further in Chapter 5.)

Sometimes, it's the discussion of the map that leads to positive changes for the team. As we mapped another physician's process, we learned that she was frustrated with the seemingly disorganized patient information she was receiving from the nurses. The nurses would see the patient first, then debrief the physician. The nurses were giving the physician what they thought was comprehensive information, but the physician only wanted to know three or four things. The rest of the information was—to the physician—annoying clutter. The physician and nurses were able to agree on the spot about what information was necessary and how to present it. Because this quickly solved a problem that had frustrated her for years, the physician became an immediate fan of the Lean process map.

Lean process mapping yielded positive change for Dr. Tassone's clinic as well. Orthopedic Center nurse Tracie Brasch says their Lean focus on the "value added" portion of the patient's visit has been sharpened in many ways. One simple point that stands out particularly is the need for patients to clearly know they have been heard and that they can have a productive consultation with the doctor.

To help ensure that patients' comments and histories have been passed along to the doctor correctly, she notes that she and her fellow nurses have asked the doctors to begin the exams by saying, "I've been told..." and then restating the information. Sometimes, the nurses will opt to talk to the doctor about these histories while in the patient exam room, so the patient clearly knows the correct information has been passed along.

"I've always felt it was all about the patient, providing the best possible care," she notes. "But now, it's easier to see the process the way the patient sees it, and it's easier to see where the value is for the patient.

By making the process work more smoothly, we feel like now we can all go that extra mile for the patient—and even leave work on time."

Creating physician flow puts the emphasis on the doctor-patient interaction, and that's a change that patients notice. Julie Pedretti tells us, "For our patients, their families, their moms, one advantage of the Lean work that we've done is that they now do feel like we know what we are doing in the overall process—they feel like their needs are being attended to, there is good communication. They truly feel like we are there to take care of them, and that's what family-centered care is all about," she says.

"Yes, we're family centered and we talk about family-centered care. But unfortunately, we've never had the tools that helped us put the patients more truly at the center. Our systems have always been around the providers, what is convenient for the physician. How does it work for our medical staff model? How does it fit in with our clinical appointment scheduling system? That's not about the patient.

"Through the Lean process, we are putting the family in the middle and we are organizing the way we do our work around them. ... The tools we've been given with Lean really put the patient in the middle. ... Lean turns everything upside down and puts the patient first. It helps us create better systems that not only make our patient families happier, but it makes our employees, our physicians happier. ... It forces us to reconfigure our resources around the patients. And that's exactly on target."

ACTION STEPS

- Analyze the scheduling template. Are appointment time slots appropriate for the practice type? Are schedule imbalances causing the clinic to run late? Trial changes to the schedule to resolve the issues you find.

- Begin to envision what a FIFO lane would look like for your physician practice.

- Observe and map the changeover process between patients. Which steps are internal and which are external? How can the internal steps be made external? Conduct quick experiments to improve changeover.

- Create a Lean process map for the physician champion's practice. Discuss what the map reveals with the team and conduct quick experiments to make improvements. Update the map to reflect the changes.

4
Step 2 – Support Physician Value-added Time

In the previous chapter, we discussed the concept of a shared resource—in this case, the physician—and how crucial it is to ensure that a shared resource is only doing value-added work. We painted the rather utopian picture of the physician going from exam room to exam room without interruption or distraction, always with the right information in hand, while the clinic staff performs changeover tasks in perfect synchronization like a well-practiced pit crew or a finely tuned orchestra.

Sounds like magic! But we all know from experience that when something looks effortless—like a physician walking into an exam room calmly, on time, and fully prepared—a lot of coordination is going on in the background. Somehow, the patient gets into the exam room, that patient's relevant information is collected and passed on, the doctor knows where that patient is, and the rest of the staff knows when to play their roles in the process. Considering that most clinics see 40, 50, or more patients every day—that's a lot of coordination enabling the physician's efficiency and success!

How can it happen?

The same need for front-line coordination occurs in manufacturing. Toyota's response was to create a team leader position for every small group or pod of workers. The team leader is someone who actually works on the team—not a manager who sits apart from the actual work—who ideally has expertise in each of the jobs performed by the team. The team leader's job is to support the front line workers by making sure they have the materials and information they need and can quickly solve problems as they arise, and by enabling them to continually improve the processes in which they operate. The team leader's position is critical to maintaining high quality standards. Unless the front line workers are supported and have the resources they need to do their jobs effectively, they are stuck being accountable for standards that are out of their control and are often reduced to working around the system.

The same scenario that caused Toyota to create a team leader position for teams assembling cars holds true for healthcare and its workers. Improvement initiatives all too often impose new standards, goals, or metrics and require people to use new tools on the job such as problem-solving techniques or new computer systems.

But, if there is no dedicated resource whose role it is to enable improvement and problem solving, those people on the front line will work around the new systems to get their jobs done the minute a problem arises. Those workarounds are not deliberate attempts to sabotage the improvements or "resist change"; rather, they are the reality of unsupported quality mandates. Faced with the choice between causing delays and problems or ignoring the new system, most healthcare providers opt for the workaround to service the patient. The Quality department or function sponsoring the improvement initiative (even Lean) is left wondering why the program became a "flavor of the month."

Remember, this is something we hear a lot. "Lean doesn't work in healthcare," a concerned executive or physician will say. "They tried it at X Hospital and after a few months had to give up." When Lean implementations fail in healthcare, one of the most common reasons is because the Lean changes were superimposed on the existing organizational structure. As long as Lean is an add-on, something extra that people are supposed to do on top of their "regular" work, the front lines will not adopt it. But, when the process changes are supported by a new organizational structure—by a new job title and responsibility specifically for the Lean system—Lean works in a profound and sustainable way.

The main organizational change that we advocate is the creation of the team leader position. In practice, this means that someone other than the physician takes charge of the clinic's operations on a very tactical level—coordinating staff schedules and scheduling templates, keeping track of where patients are and where the doctor is, and resolving the issues that interrupt patient flow. That person is the team leader.

Why not the physician? After all, we've spent so much time harping on how the physician is the leader of the clinic; why shouldn't he also take a lead role in the direction of clinic activities? Why? For the same reason that the pilot is not also the air traffic controller or that the race car driver is not also the pit crew chief. The physician's role is highly specific and requires a degree of focus and calm that is not compatible with the level of activity that the team leader directs. Further, we have found that most physicians do not want the team leader role—they would rather work with a team leader as a partner so that they are freed of decision making at the tactical level ("Where do I go next?") and can better concentrate on patient consultation and diagnosis.

Many of the team leaders we have worked with describe their philosophy at its most basic level like this: to make it easier for the physician to know what to do next. They use their knowledge of the patient mix and schedule for the day to decide which patient the physician sees next, and when in the day the physician can review billing documents or return phone calls. They may facilitate windows of time for the physician to consult with other physicians, have brief team meetings, get an answer to a question for a patient, and/or communicate any changes of which the physician may not be aware. They look at the clinic processes holistically and can help reassign resources when one function is overwhelmed. And they are a central "go to" person for problem solving and data collection. Rather than resent the time management, most physicians appreciate the clarity of direction and the clear focus.

THE TEAM LEADER IS PIVOTAL TO A LEAN TRANSFORMATION

That is certainly the case in the Orthopedic Center at Children's Hospital of Wisconsin. Nurse and team leader Lori Seubert tells us that during their Lean transformation, the creation of the team leader role was pivotal for the physicians. They quickly saw how much more smoothly the clinic ran with the team leader in place, and quite soon came to appreciate that someone was coordinating their patient schedule and workday. Within just a few weeks of the team leader introduction, one doctor joked that he would just have to cancel his clinic when the team leader took a day off.

"Creating the team lead position was key," she notes. "Suddenly everyone knew who to go to, everyone knew where to take their challenges and their successes. And most importantly, things get done."

There are many benefits of the team leader position, some tactical and obvious, others deep and transformational. On the tactical side, the team leader provides the sense that someone is "driving the bus," as Lori Seubert often says. Creating the team leader position clarifies roles and clearly puts responsibility for clinic coordination in the hands of one person. That step alone removes the feeling of chaos from a busy clinic as the team leader acts as a rudder, making sure the team is all going in the same direction. The team has a point person for questions and problems, so that issues can be resolved without causing undue wait time increases. Physicians have a point person as well, saving critical communication time and increasing time available for patient interaction. The team leader also directly influences the ability of the clinic to stay on schedule and end on time, which increases both staff and patient satisfaction.

Beyond these important day-to-day benefits, the team leader role has the power to move the Lean initiative from improvement process to team transformation, making Lean principles and a relentless focus on waste reduction and process improvement part of the team's culture. (See Figure 4.1.)

In our experience with Lean in healthcare, we have realized that the right person in the team leader role ingrains Lean in the team culture more deeply than a consultant ever could. Why? First, that team leader is part of the front line staff at the clinic, and therefore knows the clinic's demands and processes inside and out. She knows what will interrupt flow and is empowered to change it. Second, she can reinforce the use of the Lean system over an extended period of time, making sure that the improved process becomes the norm for the team and that backsliding is caught early. Finally, the team leader changes the level of discussion about clinic quality by tracking information about critical performance metrics. The simple act of collecting objective data about performance creates the ability to work collaboratively with administration and physicians on improvements, rather than placing blame or allowing personalities to take over. We'll talk much more about this shortly.

But first, let's backtrack to define what exactly a team leader is. And what exactly does a team leader do?

A team leader is typically a nurse who is given this extra level of responsibility and authority within the Lean structure, and who is compensated at a higher level or incented for the time spent as a team leader. Typically the team leader works with only one doctor, to learn and support that doctor's preferences and individual style. Other staff may rotate in the clinic, but the physician and team leader work together as a team.

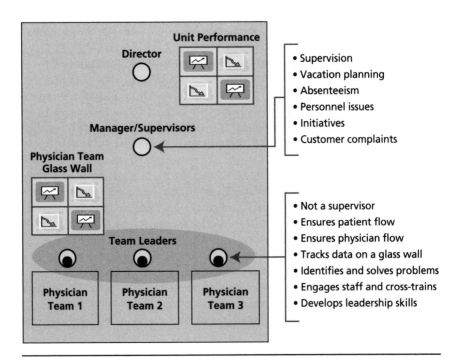

Figure 4.1 Team leader organization.

The issue of compensation is an important one, and a sticky one for many organizations. However, it's an issue that Orthopedic program administrator Terry Schwartz defined as key at Children's. In fact, she refused to move forward on creating the position until she was able to find a way to compensate the team leader accordingly.

"This was only fair, the only way to say that we recognize this role is important," she notes. Compensating the nurse for taking on the added responsibility sends the message that the organizational structure has truly changed and that the additional effort is recognized and appreciated. However, because the team leader role is often a new one for the organization, difficulty in adding a new title to an existing payroll system may bog down the Lean effort. In such cases, a little creativity goes a long way. Terry Schwartz struggled at Children's for a way to resolve this issue until one day someone happened to mention something about a position in the existing payroll system called an "Inpatient Relief Charge Nurse," which allowed nurses temporarily filling in as the charge nurse to be compensated for doing so on an hourly basis. She managed to use that payroll classification to compensate the team leaders in her clinic and did not let the payroll process or levels of bureaucracy derail either her Lean efforts or her leadership principles. Many organizations may already have people who are loosely playing parts of this role—formally or informally. In those cases, the FTEs (full time equivalent employees) may need to be incented and transferred into this role.

HOW THE TEAM LEADER "DRIVES THE BUS"

In the clinic, the team leader is responsible for maintaining the Lean system and driving it forward. This is especially important during the Lean transformation when major changes are being made and the underlying causes of delays and waste in the system are beginning to surface.

Essentially, the team leader is responsible for three clinic-based functions: clinic preparation, clinic monitoring, and clinic measurement. In addition, she's the person ultimately responsible for ensuring that processes are patient-oriented (patient advocacy) and that the clinic staff is prepared and able to "fill each other's shoes" as needed (cross-training). Each of these "bus driving" functions is vital to the success of the overall Lean effort, and of course the overall efficiency of the clinic or practice.

Clinic preparation

We'll begin with clinic preparation—it's a powerful example of how the team leader maintains the Lean system and drives it forward. The team leader is responsible for leveling the schedule at the shared resource—

the physician. Fundamentally, leveling the schedule means examining the scheduling template to be sure that the mix of patient types and the length of the appointment slots will help create flow, rather than bottlenecks. The team leader works with the physician on the template, but then takes it a step further. Each day, the team leader reviews the schedule for the next day's clinic to ensure that patients are scheduled for the right clinic (in the case of orthopedics, fractures, for example, or scoliosis) and that each is scheduled for the appropriate length of time.

Because an improperly scheduled patient creates an unavoidable problem for the clinic, this "scrubbing" of the schedule is invaluable to patient flow. In this case, the team leader is supporting the front line workers by removing potential problems before they disrupt clinic flow. Patients also benefit from this preventive step—they are seen in the right clinic without unnecessary delays and frustrations.

An in-depth review of the schedule also allows the team leader to make sure adequate support resources are available to deal with the expected volume of patients, thereby removing another common source of wait times and chaos in the clinic. Particularly in outpatient care, it is often difficult to assess how many resources are needed for a given volume of patients. The expertise the team leader develops over time by reviewing the schedule is valuable to the clinic.

The result of all of this preparation is that preventable problems and sources of waste are taken out of the system. The team is not surprised in a busy fractures clinic with 10-minute appointment slots by a scoliosis patient who requires a 30-minute consultation. Bottlenecks at casting or radiology do not develop because there are enough people to handle that day's patient load. The physician does not waste time looking for information that should be included in the charts. In short, the team leader's preparation ensures that the clinic can achieve flow.

Clinic monitoring

With the "clinic preparation" work done and the schedule leveled, the team leader focuses on the actual operation of the clinic or practice, or the flow. During the clinic day, the team leader's goal is to ensure that every time the physician enters an exam room, the patient is ready for him.

To do this, the team leader must stay up to the moment on the status of each patient in the clinic and direct staff and resources to the specific needs of the individual patient. For example, if the team leader in a busy fractures clinic sees that five of eight patients in the clinic are in x-ray, she can direct other resources to radiology to alleviate the bottleneck.

When the physician enters the exam room, all of the changeover tasks must already have been successfully completed. If the patient has to have a cast removed or x-rays taken prior to an exam, those steps must be completed. Seeing patients is the value-added task for the physician;

she must never walk into an exam room to find a patient who is not yet ready to be seen. Through clinic preparation and continual monitoring, the team leader supports that value-added time.

Clinic measurement

Finally, the team leader is responsible for allowing the staff to take a periodic "step back from the bus" and look at the larger efficiency picture. The team leader maintains a "glass wall" of metrics that are important to the physician, the clinic staff, and the patient.

A glass wall is a bulletin board in the clinic where graphs of key metrics are posted for all clinic staff to see. (See Figure 4.2.) The term glass wall refers to the transparency of the data. The graphs for performance metrics are posted and updated by the team leader, making the clinic's performance transparent to all those who view the graphs. She uses the data to identify problems that surface repeatedly in the clinic and set goals for continuous improvement.

Children's Quality Data Management (QDM) team created a database for glass wall data collection that has flexibility in the field headings so that each clinic can collect data about the metrics most important to it. Now, the team leaders collect data and send the sheet to QDM at the end of each week. Then that data is entered into the database, where it is accessible to a wide audience.

The benefit to this system is that the team leader owns the data and can trust its integrity. Thanks to this database, the team leaders have faith in the numbers they get. They own the data and they trust it, which provides a good foundation for data-driven decision making.

For example, a team leader may learn from a physician that the most critical metrics are clinic end times, clinic errors (such as missing radiology films), and patient volume by injury type or complexity. She would collect ongoing data to see trends of issues, set joint goals with the working team, and coordinate improvement activities. For example, the data may indicate a problem—perhaps the clinic consistently runs over—for which the team leader is able to set an improvement goal and begin a problem solving process.

The old adage, "what gets measured gets managed," is certainly true. The simple act of tracking key performance indicators focuses the staff's attention on them and leads to improvement. Nurse and team leader Lori Seubert notes that the glass wall engages everyone on a fundamentally different level.

"The doctors were getting emotionally involved because a lot of things were problematic and the doctors would mention these problems. But during the busy clinic day, it all would kind of be forgotten. Now, we can collect data over months and actually see our progress. That's very powerful" she says.

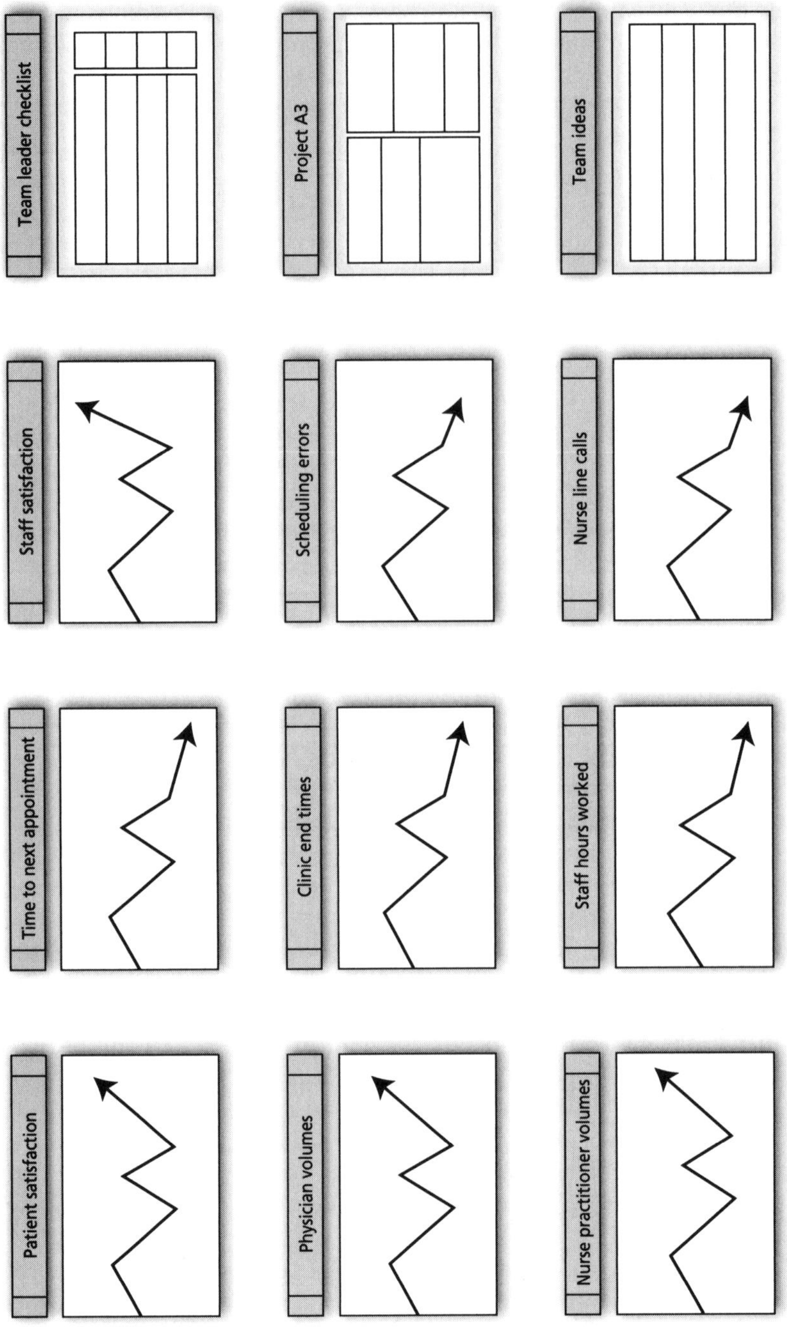

Figure 4.2 Physician glass wall.

"This tracking is visible and it's a clear communication path. These are numbers. They are concrete. The numbers are the numbers. That's how it is. We had ten scheduling errors and we got down to five. That takes hard work. And now it's visible and it's recognized. Everyone can see it and get a snapshot of what's going on."

Patient advocacy

The team leader maintains the Lean system by using and developing processes that are patient focused. She is the point person for continuing to drive out waste to reduce patient wait times and improve patient satisfaction. She has the responsibility to keep the patient's point of view in mind whenever processes are changed or improved.

For example, a team leader may help develop a short survey to collect data from a given set of patients at the end of their visits to monitor trends and opportunities in patient satisfaction. A team leader may also look ahead to ensure patients are correctly scheduled and phone patients to remind them of information needed for the clinic visit. Or, she may help manage patient needs within the clinic, coordinating appointments with other departments, for example.

Cross training of the clinic team

Cross training is a great way to build added capacity into the clinic staff, so that in busy times team members who are not overbooked can help those who are. Team leaders manage cross training programs, maintaining training records and ensuring that those who are cross-trained can proficiently perform the new tasks. Team leaders can also choose personnel for cross training who can handle added responsibility so that additional training becomes an earned reward and job enrichment.

For example, the Clinic Assistant in the Orthopedic Center received training from one of the team leaders to remove dressings for patients who visit the clinic after surgery. Other team members received training from the physical therapy department about teaching children how to walk with crutches. This particular example not only provided a job enrichment opportunity for the staff members, but also eliminated a walk to the Physical Therapy department for the patients and their families. Cross training is a tangible benefit of the team leader role. The staff appreciates the opportunity to learn new skills and participate in new ways in the care process, and the practice can more easily reallocate resources when there's a backlog.

"One of the top problems identified for improvement was nurses having to wait for physicians to return calls or visit so they could update the physicians on changes in their patients' conditions that could affect treatment and discharge plans. Resolving the problem could result in more timely communication, shorter hospital stays, and reduced inefficiencies such as having to make repeated calls to physicians and search for nurses to take the returned calls."

From "Improving Communication with Bedside Video Rounding" by Peachy B. Hain, MSN, RN et al, *Journal of Nursing*, November 2009, Vol. 109, No. 11 Supplement)

HOW TO CHOOSE AND DEVELOP EFFECTIVE LEAN TEAM MEMBERS

A good team leader candidate is a nurse who has shown interest in developing beyond his or her current role, who has good relationships with the practice team, who knows the practice's processes and supporting functions well, and who works well with the physician champion. Team leaders need training, coaching, and support, especially as they begin in the role. The team leader position requires a different set of skills; we have found these competencies to be especially vital:

- **Data management:** The glass wall is the engine that drives the team leader's problem solving and continuous improvement capability in the clinic. To effectively manage the glass wall, the team leader must identify metrics that are relevant to the practice team, collect data related to those metrics, and graph it. After the glass wall is established, the team leader can involve other team members in the data collection to encourage ownership of improvements efforts, but the primary responsibility for data collection and graphing belongs to the team leader. She may need additional skill development in creating graphs and understanding variation.

- **Problem Solving:** The problem solving process is a great developmental opportunity for team leaders. In order to do it well, they must use the data they are collecting on the glass wall to identify the next high-priority problem to solve, solicit feedback from the team about root causes and possible solutions, and trial the solutions in the practice. All of this takes a foundation in basic problem solving tools, plus team management skills and a healthy dose of interpersonal savvy. We use the A3 form to help organize the problem solving process (see the Appendix for a copy).

- **Understanding of Lean Systems Principles:** Team leaders are responsible for managing the Lean system and continuing to drive waste out of the clinic processes. They need training in the seven wastes, flow, value stream mapping, standard work, and 5S, among other principles. Introducing a principle and working projects to put that principle into practice most effectively accomplishes this training. For example, a team leader may attend a short training session on the principle of 5S and then lead a 5S project in the clinic.

- **Interpersonal Skills:** Team leaders impact everyone else in the clinic. They will be much more successful if they are equipped with an understanding of interpersonal dynamics, consensus building, and conflict management.

The managers of team leaders must recognize the critical role they play in the success of the team leader position. It is not enough to create the role—it must be supported. Specifically, managers of team leaders must:

1. Take a personal interest in the metrics on the glass wall, express the expectation that the team leader will learn to collect and graph the data (with initial help, if needed), and encourage the physician and the staff to review the data and offer improvement ideas.

2. Provide support for the team leader's problem solving efforts. As a manager, your role is to continuously challenge the team leader and the team by pointing out trends in the data, probing, asking for deeper involvement through problem solving, and aiding the team with goal setting. In short, ensure that the glass wall serves its role as driver of the problem solving process.

3. Let go of some of the day-to-day management of the practice and let the team leader develop in her role of process owner for the clinic. You may need to establish guidelines and boundaries with the team leader, but then be ready to be less involved with daily decision making.

The team leader becomes the person who "drives the bus" in a busy clinic environment. Although it's a busy, demanding position, our experience has shown it proves its value on many Lean levels.

"This renewed my whole sense of value in myself," explains Children's Orthopedic Center nurse and team leader Tracie Brasch. "I'm not just following a doctor into the room and standing by in case he needs me. It gave me a boost professionally, after 23 years as a nurse at Children's Hospital. I feel more respected. I feel more valued.

It's enjoyable to work with people who are all of like mind, where the important thing is providing the best care for the patients—while still taking care of ourselves."

She adds: "Of course, everyone has to be ready to change. But it's nice to reach a point where we all value each other's opinions. We may feel differently about some things, but now we have the tools to come together. It's all a tremendous sense of accomplishment at the end of the day."

ACTION STEPS

- Identify (and incent) the team leader to work specifically with the physician champion.

- Provide training and development for the team leader in the areas of data collection, problem solving, Lean principles, and interpersonal skills.

- Begin to define the team leader responsibilities in the areas of clinic preparation, monitoring and measurement, patient advocacy, and cross training.

- Begin a glass wall.

- Review the glass wall data with the team to identify improvement opportunities.

- Continue to review and define the team leader role as clinic operations change and improve.

5
Step 3 – Visually Communicate Patient Status

Now it's time to create your clinic "crystal ball." With this success step, I'm going to describe a simple, low-tech tool that will empower everyone on your healthcare team to quickly see how things are progressing, what steps to take now, and what to expect next. It's a tool that's so transformative that nurses in Dr. Tassone's clinic at Children's Hospital describe it as their crystal ball and say implementing it marked a clear turning point on their Lean journey.

First some background: The Lean concept of visual communication uses markers, signals, and signs to create a system of autonomous control that requires the least possible supervision. The system communicates the status of a given process to the entire working team so everyone can tell what's in progress, what's working, and where the problems are. It's designed to facilitate the transfer of important information as quickly as possible so corrective action can begin as soon as possible, by the experts performing the work.

Lean recognizes that sharing important information visually has several significant benefits and goals:

- Information is shared with people who can make a real-time difference in the outcome.

- The same real-time information is available to everyone on the team, no matter what their individual role or place in the system hierarchy.

- It promotes a "self-service" environment in which staff is able to take away the information needed to make decisions on what to do next or what to improve.

- Everyone on the team knows how their role fits into the overall process and that their actions and tasks have a meaning.

- Because it is designed to be visible over longs distances, visual communication saves wasted motion for the staff.

Remember: A key component of Lean is precisely that it is team-focused and empowering. That's part of the beauty of visual communication. It provides essential information and performance feedback to *all* team members, regardless of title or rank. All team members have the same information for problem solving, process improvement, and decision-making.

This is vital to any Lean transformation. And it helps explain why, in many ways, this step has proven to be the most transformative for the doctors, nurses, and healthcare workers in the Lean process. With this step, so many of the pieces I've been detailing suddenly come together so the processes click and work. Conversely, however, it's also a step that often draws the most vocal opposition because it requires visible and obvious change in how things are done.

"In the beginning, I couldn't see how this was going to help us," explains Orthopedic nurse Tracie Brasch. "It felt like it was just going to be *more* work. How could this make us more efficient? Now, it's like, duh, this really works. But back then, I couldn't see how it was going to change our old ways."

The key is this: In an environment with well-designed visual communication, people can make decisions about what actions to take next more easily and with less waste.

VISUAL COMMUNICATION IN HEALTHCARE: THE CLINIC STATUS BOARD

So, what exactly is visual communication and how does it work in a Lean healthcare transformation?

At its most basic level, simple forms of visual communication in everyday life tell us whether a checkout lane at the grocery store is open, when to stop for a school bus, or when our cars need maintenance.

In the clinic or practice environment, visual communication will help us "drive the bus" by answering the most basic question physicians face during their clinic days—a question that ultimately determines whether our shared resource, the physician, is able to achieve the flow we described earlier.

The question: *How do I know what to do next?*

That might sound obvious, or a bit too basic. But think about the physician's job without visual communication. Without visual communication, a physician comes out of an exam room and does not have a clear picture of who is next in line to be seen. Sometimes a clinic assistant might act as a traffic director and tell the physician which room is next. Or perhaps he goes into a room because he sees charts outside the exam room indicating that a patient is waiting. Sometimes patients come out of exam rooms to question the wait time and check their own status. In all of these cases, the physician is either guessing what the next priority is or can be easily taken off course by unscheduled activities. The physician is dependent on verbal updates about patient status—updates that may or may not be current.

The same confusion impacts the rest of the clinic staff as well. If the nurses, residents, and physician's assistants do not know the status of each patient in the clinic, there is unnecessary checking, delay, and frustration in the process. These are the wastes that increase patient wait times, lower patient satisfaction, and create stress for staff as well.

And so to adapt Lean visual communication tools to the clinic, we created the clinic status board that addresses these issues by making patient status visible to the entire clinic team. (See Figure 5.1.) It is a low-tech answer with powerful results. The status board tells the staff where in the clinic each patient is located. It is simply a whiteboard with taped columns for each process step and a marker and a magnet for each patient.

As the patient moves through the care process, the team leader moves the magnet into the appropriate column. At a glance, the team leader (and the rest of the clinic staff) knows exactly where the bottlenecks and waits are, what must be done next, and where the physician's next priority is.

Before we go into greater detail about the patient status board, I think it's important to note that in the case of Dr. Tassone's clinic in the Orthopedic Center at Children's Hospital (like almost any other environment), they did have some forms of visual communication related to patient status before our Lean transformation. In their case, the staff had a whiteboard that was supposed to communicate information about patient status, but it was not comprehensive or reliable. The tool was in need of its own Lean transformation.

"The whiteboard used to be: 'This patient has arrived and this is the doctor they're going to see and the time of their appointment. And that's it," says Tracie Brasch, the nurse. "We knew they were here, somewhere. But were they now in x-ray? Or in the cast room? Back in the waiting room? Where were they?"

The Lean process transformed the whiteboard into a clinic status board that conveyed the information staff truly needed to make decisions about what to handle next. The process works like this:

- As a fracture patient progresses through the fracture clinic, a magnet with the patient's name written on it represents that patient on the clinic status board. (Some clinics add the appointment time and a color code for new or follow up patients to the magnet as well.)

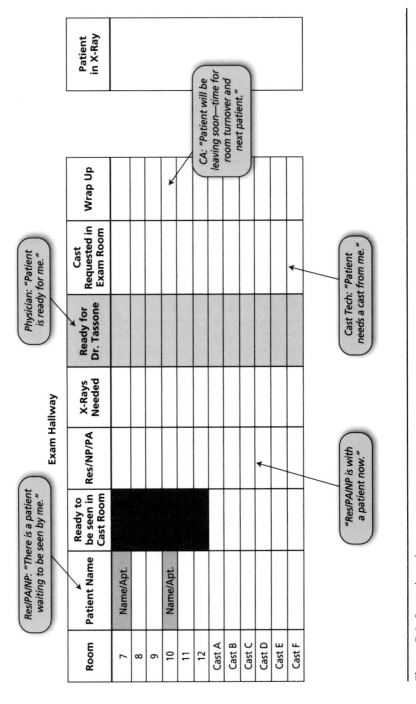

Figure 5.1 Status board.

- Any member of the clinic team can move the patient's name along the status board, but it is the team leader's special responsibility to know the status of each patient and know where the physician is at all times during the clinic. Using the status board as a visual guide, the team leader tells the physician, for example, that exam room 2 is next, followed by exam room 4. The physician does not have to decide where to go next, leaving it to the team leader to direct flow through the clinic.

Key to achieving this flow is ensuring that the patient is not moved to the "MD" column of the status board unless all changeover steps have been completed. The physician's value-added time is increased when she presents only to those patients' rooms who are actually ready. The status board is constantly monitored and updated by the team leader; it is the tool the team leader uses to provide direction and increase the physician's available time for patient interaction.

When both the status board and the team leader are in place, the physician is like a pilot, free to focus 100 percent on the task at hand, while the air traffic controller (the team leader) uses the radar (the status board) to oversee the larger picture.

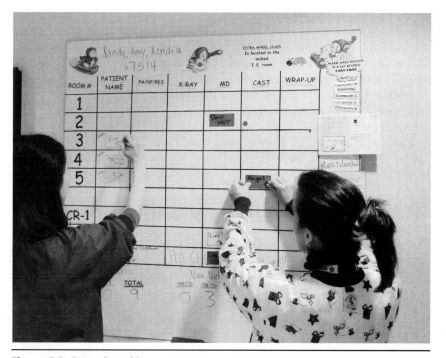

Figure 5.2 Status board in use.

WHY DOES VISUAL COMMUNICATION WORK SO EFFECTIVELY?

Visual communication using such a status board allows the board itself to become a trigger for the next work in the process to begin. When a patient moves to the next status column, the person doing the work automatically assumes duties without being told. If the patient is ready to be seen for casting, the cast technicians are aware that a patient is waiting. If the physician finishes with the patient and moves him or her to the wrap up column, the nurse can be available to answer final questions and the clinic assistant can be ready to quickly turn over the room and get the next patient in.

The status board also creates the FIFO lanes we discussed earlier and ensures that the patients are seen in the order in which they are ready. Visually communicating patient status removes the possibility that some wait longer than others simply because no one knows where they are.

That status board also reduces waste of motion. Just as we can see a stoplight from 500 feet away and make a decision to stop or go, the visual board can communicate the status of the entire clinic from anywhere within the clinic area, helping each team member prioritize tasks to support patient and provider flow.

Finally, the status board also provides a powerful visual image of the clinic operations. If the team leader sees a cluster of patient magnets in the casting column, for example, she can reallocate resources and alleviate the bottleneck. The visual summary of clinic activity is invaluable; in fact, it is why the nurses compare the status board to a "clinic crystal ball."

"The board also invests everyone in how the clinic is running," notes Dr. Tassone, "from the MA to the residents to myself. Having that information right there in the middle of everything reminds people what they need to be doing. They can tell if they aren't seeing as many people in clinic as they should. They can tell how many people are waiting for a room. They can tell where I am and start to anticipate my availability to guide their next steps."

THE PATIENT STATUS BOARD IN ACTION

At Dr. Tassone's clinic, the clinic status board was truly a transformational tool in the Lean process. It became a good barometer of ownership of the Lean system—if a particular person didn't use it, that became noticeable very quickly. And it was the most visible change in the clinic, the one that still is most often shown off when visitors come to the clinic. In some ways, it has become the symbol of the team's ownership and cohesion.

Even Dr. Ramesh Sachdeva, the Children's Hospital corporate vice president and chief quality officer, noticed what a sense of transformation came over the clinic with the clinic status board.

"I will never forget when I was walking through the Orthopedic clinic and there was the whiteboard—and the ownership was fantastic," Dr. Sachdeva recalls. "They all owned it. The nurses, the physicians, they owned it. They all felt that this is their whiteboard. It is not the consultant's whiteboard; it is my whiteboard. It's that level of ownership that drove the excitement that ends up translating the ownership to the people in the front lines."

However, this sense of ownership did not happen overnight or without effort. Nurse Beth Wahlquist says the use of the status board generated the most vocal opposition to the whole Lean process. Until its implementation, much of the transformation was more "talk" and the status board required a very visible change in behavior. As she explains: "At first, the clinic team thought, 'We don't need all these slots. The whiteboard could be simpler.'"

However, the reluctant people got on board simply because it didn't go away—and so they stuck with it until it became a habit.

That happened in large part because program administrator Terry Schwartz made it a clear priority to get everybody on board on this stage of the process. Once she saw the benefits of the whiteboard for Dr. Tassone's clinic, she felt that this change was essential for every physician's practice. She cleared her schedule, we created a second whiteboard for another physician's practice, and she literally stood next to the whiteboards for the first three days to make sure everyone used it consistently. (This is also a good example of how deep analysis of one physician's practice can sometimes lead to immediate and obvious changes for other physicians.)

"Essentially, I was there saying: This is important. We need to do this," she explains. "I was not just walking away."

Without that administrative presence and commitment, the change to using the whiteboard uniformly might not have happened—and the whole Lean transformation process could have been derailed rather than picking up speed and supporters.

Although staff at first felt that the board was too detailed, in the time since undertaking the initial Lean transformation, the clinic has actually added more detail to the board as an attempt to communicate the full picture to the physician. There are now yellow name magnets for follow-up patients, red magnets for new patients, blue dots for the cast column if the cast is being put on, red dots for cast off. Other more specialized magnets indicate where the films are (on the reader or the computer screen) and medical abbreviations. Further, the name magnet also includes the appointment time and the initials of the person who has responsibility for the first step (Physician's Assistant, Nurse Practitioner, or Resident). When a patient is moved to the Wrap Up column and the physician is completely finished with her, the name is crossed through to indicate that the physician doesn't have to worry about that one.

The main goal of all that information on the board is to keep the physician up to date or, more accurately, to keep the people telling the physician what to do next up to date. Now there are several visual communication tools that the physician uses to know where to go next: the flags outside the door (a red flag means go here next), the names on the board in the MD column, the countdown number on the board, and the team leader directing traffic.

In fact, to describe the level of efficiency achieved with the clinic status board, I'll tell you about a visit I made to the clinic several months after our Lean transformation. I visited the clinic to track and observe processes. Only I quickly became bored—really bored. I thought I was there to see the seasonal rush of patients and to experience the swell of activity that an annual volume of 24,000 patients could bring. Instead, I sat on a stool and watched the surgeon walk out of an exam room, get direction from his team leader, and walk into another exam room. Occasionally he dictated a file or stopped to chat with the rest of the staff. His team leader, Lori Seubert, updated the whiteboard continuously, moving magnets depending on where patients were in the clinic, but that was the extent of "activity."

At the end of the afternoon, I was surprised to realize that more than 40 patients had been seen in just over three hours. "Forty?" I thought. "Where were the crises? Where was the running around, the heroic efforts?" There were none. What I witnessed was a focused, calm work environment in which everyone had access to patient status information, no one had to ask for direction about the next priority, and no patients got lost in the system.

The clinic had already established physician flow and had created the team leader role. But the key to getting the most out of those two important changes was its use of visual communication. Remember: the status board is the tool the team leader uses to keep the patients flowing in the clinic and to ensure the shared resource—the physician—is scheduled as effectively as possible. Without the powerful simplicity of the status board, the team leader's job would be nearly impossible.

More about how Dr. Tassone's staff uses the board

The clinic assistant will note on the whiteboard that the patient's images are available for viewing. In the clinic, they have a laminated card titled "On Reader" with magnets on the back. This is placed in that individual patient's 'x-ray' column of the whiteboard. In addition, they have laminated magnetic cards labeled with words they use repeatedly for whiteboard use.

If the patient has brought x-ray, MRI, or CT-scan images that are stored on a disc, then the clinic assistant will load the disc in a computer to be viewed on the dual monitoring screens. The clinic assistant will note this with a laminated designator card on the whiteboard in the appropriate patient's area. Next, the clinic assistant makes sure the patient's name magnet is located by the correct exam room number on the whiteboard, that the chart is located in the chart holder bin located right outside of the patient's exam room, and that the patient is tracked electronically to the correct exam room number.

New patients, who require more time in the exam room, have red magnets next to their names. Follow-up patients have yellow magnets, giving the physician a quick visual cue about the time requirements for the day. Further, the clinic assistant created laminated magnetic cards with short descriptions such as, "Pins Out," "Suture Removal," and "Range of Motion" to summarize for the team what each patient's visit requires.

Finally, the clinic assistant records the number of patients booked for the day at the top of the status board and counts down as each patient is added to the status board throughout the day. This has proven to be a powerful visual metric for the physicians, who are often not fully aware of how many patients they have booked for a particular clinic. That awareness can lead to an adjustment of scheduling templates or protocols to prevent chronic overbooking and late-ending clinics. The physician can also use the "countdown" number to prioritize patients: If there are two or more in the "MD" column, the physician knows to see the patient with the higher number first, assuring the FIFO lane works.

IF VISUAL COMMUNICATION WORKS SO WELL, WHY NOT START THERE?

Visual communication is tangible and concrete and it's often the place where Lean teams want to begin. After all, hanging a new whiteboard in the hallway is relatively easy and more appealing work than reviewing scheduling templates or battling the status quo to create team leaders. Yet, it is success step number three in our list for some compelling reasons:

- First, if you have not created physician flow by scheduling the physician as a shared resource and reducing changeover time, the status board will only serve to highlight chaos. Although there is value to making process problems highly visible, the status board itself does nothing to fundamentally change a flawed process. So, the team gets the message loud and clear that the process is broken—quite the opposite of the motivating, empowering tool the status board is intended to be.

- Second, if the team leader position has not been created to provide responsibility for patient flow in general and the status board specifically, the board will quickly fall into disuse. The status board must have an owner to keep it up to date and ensure that the information it provides is timely and relevant. The team leader is an essential part of making visual communication work in the clinic. When those pieces are in place to enable a fundamentally different process, creating the board provides not only visual communication of patient status, but a visual transformation of the clinic as well.

In a Lean transformation, visual communication goes far beyond simple boards or markers. It becomes the tool that ties all the pieces of the Lean system together into a cohesive whole. The status board provides the information the team leader needs to direct clinic activities and support the physician's value-added time. That information also empowers all staff members to respond to bottlenecks and crises that arise. And it allows the staff to see how their roles and tasks—which we have previously demoted to "changeover"—fit together to directly impact that overall goal of minimizing patient wait times.

That information and insight has a remarkable effect on the clinic staff: It makes them a team. They have a clear and shared goal. They know how they help achieve that goal. They have role clarity and clear direction. They have a knowledgeable leader "driving the bus."

"This is definitely one of the key components toward the success that we have had," notes Dr. Tassone. "This brings Lean to the forefront of everyone's mind every time they step out of a patient room and right before they go in. It also gives the provider the oversight of everything that is happening in their clinic at all times: where people are, how long people have been waiting, how many people, and so on. I believe this was a significant component in reducing wait times for the patients."

And once the team begins to see the benefits of making communication visual, more opportunities to use the tool become apparent. For example, a basket for patient intake paperwork placed at the front desk acts as a visual queue for the clinic assistant, indicating that the next patient is ready to come back to an exam room. Making this kind of communication visual, rather than verbal, takes potential errors of miscommunication out of the system. Lean practitioners call this kind of visual control a "kanban," which shows the movement of "material" through the system.

ACTION STEPS

- Define the patient stages for your physician practice.

- Design your clinic status board to represent those stages. Trial the design before making permanent columns on the board.

- Brainstorm common conditions that can be easily represented on the clinic status board, as well as other information relevant to the practice that can be summarized on the board.

- Clearly define who is responsible for updating the clinic status board.

6

Step 4 – Standardize Everyone's Work

A place for everything and everything in its place...a well designed job for everyone and everyone improving their job.

That's the basic idea behind standard work, which comes along at this stage of the Lean transformation process for a reason. It's a concept that's a bit difficult to understand, a bit cumbersome to execute, even a bit counterintuitive to the Lean process. But it's also a key step on your Lean journey, and you'll want to resist any temptation to skip on by. Remember the people who say Lean cannot work in the healthcare environment? They're the people who most likely skipped this Lean tool.

I'll define standard work in much greater detail as I describe what you'll need to do to complete this success step. But to begin: standard work is a tool of Lean that provides process stability and a mechanism for formal process improvement. It is based on an important underlying premise of Lean: that the process defines the outcome. If your process is not clearly defined, the outcome is left to chance. With standard work, everyone clearly defines their own processes.

That sounds complicated, but it simply means that you need a clearly defined process in order to do your job efficiently and effectively, and you need to re-evaluate this frequently in order to capture improvements. In other words: a well-defined job for everyone, and everyone improving their job.

Standard work is a document, developed by individual staff members, that captures the particular steps and activities that he or she completes (in the case of healthcare, for providing patient care). It describes one person and one job. A standard work document includes:

- Main process steps (also known as work elements)

- Key points to ensure safety and/or quality of the task, reminders, and tips for success under those steps

- Sequence or order of steps
- Supplies or forms needed to complete the job
- The time it takes to complete each step
- A layout diagram of where each step is completed, if applicable

WHY STANDARD WORK IN HEALTHCARE?

In our Lean work in healthcare environments, we have observed that patients may get inconsistent service depending on what day of the week they visit and who they interact with at the hospital, clinic, or practice. Two secretaries on two different days at the same clinic, for example, may greet the patient differently (not such a big deal), ask for information in a different sequence (not great, but patients can handle this), or give conflicting answers to a patient's question (now we're heading for trouble).

Patients have, in many ways, come to expect this. They know people do things differently. But imagine what this can mean for a hospital system trying to create consistent service standards. Imagine trying to train a new person with nothing written down about what to do or how to do a particular job in an efficient manner. And imagine not understanding how your role impacts everyone else's role on a patient care team, or how all of it impacts the actual quality of patient care.

And so this is important: *standard work provides a way to document the patient care process.* Let's examine this more closely. Everyone who interacts with the patient performs a role in the overall patient care. Chances are these individuals need supplies (such as sutures). They need to know what the patient needs (communication of the need from a doctor or someone overseeing the care of the patient). They need to know what steps to take to make the best and most efficient experience for the patient. They need to know what questions they can expect from the patient and how to answer them. And they need to know how to communicate to the next provider in line when they finish, so patients aren't waiting longer than they have to.

Looking at it this way, standard work identifies what to do with each patient from beginning to end, including communication to the rest of the staff. How does this get done without standard work in place? It typically gets done simply based on the knowledge and experience that each person has. That may work perfectly. Or, more likely, it may involve waste (such as sutures being located far away). It may involve unclear communication regarding the needs of the patient. Or there may be better and more efficient ways of doing the job.

To give just one simple example: Dr. Tassone's administrative assistant, Amy Ricely, is the person responsible for scheduling his surgeries. But before this stage of the Lean transformation, she never really understood how scheduling decisions affected the actual flow of the surgery day.

"I learned things I never knew before, in five years of doing this job," she notes. "When we sat down and I understood how the surgery room flows, I could see important things about scheduling: that it helps to group similar surgeries together, that it's best to schedule the lengthiest cases first. Little things that I never would have thought twice about and things that I just didn't hear about.

"When you learn how something functions, it makes you more aware and you can do your job better," she says. "And this opens up communication 100 percent."

Standard work is sometimes confused with other documents that provide information about a job.

- Standard work is *not* a job description, which defines a job's main accountabilities and how that job fits into the larger organization.

- Standard work is *not* an overall process description, which would include more than one person and the handoffs between functions.

- Standard work is *not* a standard operating procedure, which shows work in a great level of detail and often includes OSHA references and so on.

Standard work can take many different forms depending on the organization, but all have the same elements: main process steps, work elements, time, needed supplies, and layout. Most important, it is created and updated by the people doing the job. (Remember, Lean is "pulled," not "pushed." It cannot simply be driven from the top down.)

THE BENEFITS OF CREATING STANDARD WORK

I hope it's becoming clear that without standard work, frustration may be the only truly predictable outcome at the end of the day!

The most fundamental reason for creating standard work is that it provides a mechanism for improving the process. Process improvement starts with analyzing what you actually do to complete your required tasks. The mere process of looking critically at your own work and writing down the steps makes you start thinking. It gets the wheels turning. You notice things you never realized before. You look at things differently. For example, if you've had training in the seven wastes and principles of Lean (see appendix) before starting to create standard work, you might immediately start to see the wastes in your own job. You might see ways to do things more effectively. You might even uncover things that don't need to be done.

The act of writing standard work also begins to expose opportunities where errors might occur. There is a methodology in Lean known as error-proofing, or poke-yoke. *Poke-yoke* is a Japanese word translated as "fail-safing" or "mistake-proofing." Poke-yoke helps team members work easily, and at the same time it eliminates troubles associated with defects, safety, mistakes in operation, and so on without requiring the person's undue attention.

As workers document their own tasks, opportunities for errors and safety become obvious. The creativity of the team members is tapped to come up with ways of avoiding errors. You know you can't fit a diesel nozzle in a regular automobile gasoline tank; it is designed that way to prevent that error. A simple example of this in the clinic environment might involve color-coding patient charts for different physicians or color-coding new versus follow-up patients in the chart preparation process.

The standard work document also becomes the place to capture improvements. If there is nothing that defines the work method, then there is no way to improve it on a systemic level. One person—one nurse or PA, for example—might come up with a more efficient way to do his or her job. But without standard work documents that define how the job is done, there is no place to capture a change. This is what we mean by capturing "best practices." So, although it is sometimes counterintuitive, it is precisely standardization that allows for easier improvement.

By creating these standard work documents, you'll also uncover resource imbalances and places where people have either too much or too little time to complete their tasks. In the process of capturing the time needed for each job in the clinic, you may realize that a resource has time on his or her hands at certain points of the day. Once you are aware that resources are imbalanced, tasks can be reassigned to correct the imbalance, or that time can be put to good use in cross-training.

Standard work helps define what the tasks are that keep the clinic operating smoothly; knowing how long it takes to complete each task helps managers ensure that no resource is overloaded or under-utilized. It can also help a manager determine how many resources are needed for a given schedule and answer such questions as these: What's the work content of a secretary on a busy afternoon? How many cast techs are needed for a clinic in July?

Finally, standard work ensures that handoffs and interactions among staff go smoothly. Remember: a busy clinic or practice comprises five or six different roles that interact with the patient separately or together to provide care. In most cases, these people have not been trained together; they are at different levels in the organization, they have different perspectives, and they have varying expectations of each other. They are the secretaries at the front desk, clinic assistants who room the patients, nurses who prepare charts and care for patients, PA's who conduct initial assessments, physicians who are the target for everything, cast techs, and radiology techs. As the patient interfaces with each role, there are handoffs and the transfer of information.

In the absence of standardization, each person in the clinic will develop an individual method of working and everyone will do things his or her own way. Of course, this is not a willful attempt to cause problems; it is simply the result of having to get the job done in the absence of an agreed-upon method. But it becomes more complicated because some will not like the methods coworkers are using. Perhaps one person prefers the paperwork assembled in one way, or a particular level of detail in notes, or a particular method of casting. Unless open confrontation is part of your clinic's culture, people may begin to form cliques with others who prefer to work together. On those days, things run smoothly. However, substitute someone else into the mix and problems arise. This kind of underground conflict can lead to ongoing personality clashes and higher stress levels among team members.

The process of creating standard work clarifies roles and expectations, provides a forum for discussions about methods and improvement, and removes the root causes of many kinds of workplace conflict.

Finally, standard work makes training new employees easier. In many organizations, on-the-job training means following an experienced worker around for a couple of days to "learn the ropes." The new employee is supposed to observe the experienced worker and then do things the same way. Problems occur, however, when that experienced worker has a different way of doing tasks than other people in the same position, passes along inaccurate or incomplete direction to the new employee, or does the job incorrectly.

But if the job has been defined through standard work, new employees can read the standard work document and use it to observe the experienced worker. The trainer, in turn, can walk through the standard work as he or she demonstrates the task and explain critical steps or outcomes to the new employee. Using standard work as a tool for new employee training ensures that valuable process knowledge will not be lost, and that turnover in the clinic will not mean a return to chaotic work practices.

As we have introduced the concept of standard work in the various Lean areas, the teams have brainstormed the following list of benefits to the process:

- Standard work helps provide consistent patient service.
- Standard work removes interpersonal barriers by clarifying staff roles.
- Standard work helps us anticipate and prevent potential error.
- Standard work gives us a process to schedule the right patients in the right clinics.
- Standard work ensures that new people are trained on the same page.
- Standard work ensures that high quality is built into our processes and expected by everyone.
- Standard work allows both staff and administration to agree on the right resource levels.
- Standard work eliminates the seven wastes of Lean.

PROCESS FOR CREATING STANDARD WORK

To complete this success step, everyone on your healthcare pilot team will be creating a standard work document as described in detail here. As you clearly define what must happen to make the clinic flow and reduce wait times, it translates into each member of the team defining her part of the job.

For example, the team leader's standard work may include ensuring that computers are turned on, that patient charts are prepped, and that the entire team is set for the day. The medical assistant or clinic assistant may make sure that each of the exam rooms is set with needed supplies and forms. All this preparation must be done on a consistent basis to eliminate surprises. During the clinic, as the day begins, staff members interacting with the patient must communicate before and after they see a patient. As needs come up during the day, the team leader may be charged with solving a specific patient problem while the rest of the team keeps moving. The physician may need to get a debriefing before walking into the patient room, every time, to ensure no overlap in questions.

As Lean expands in a department or a clinic, these standard work documents will be shared among people doing the same job (for example, nurses or casting technicians). You may find certain practices among nurses for example, that become the standard because they are efficient and create a better experience for the patient. Then you'll define "best practices" and systematically integrate process improvements into the workplace.

So let us move on to the actual process for creating standard work documents. Standard work begins with individuals writing the steps they go through to perform their required tasks in the left hand column of the standard work form. At first, there is no need to include work elements, to indicate whether the step is value-added, or to determine how long it takes to complete. There is also no need for special computer programs or complicated formats; simply capture the steps using a copy of the form and a pencil. (See Table 6.1.)

Because clinics have more than one person performing each job, the next step is to compare the first drafts, look for obvious areas for improvement, and agree on a basic process among all those who perform that job. This step often involves some negotiation and compromise and is best done with a "let's try it and see" attitude. Nothing is set permanently on paper, and changes and improvements can be easily made. Once a draft process is determined, the team can jointly decide to revise it.

Once the main steps are agreed upon, it is time to gather the additional detail that the form captures. The people doing the jobs are the ones who should gather the information about work elements, times, and layouts. Further, that information should be gleaned through direct observation and measurement as the job is being done, rather than through estimation in a conference room. Clinic team members can carry a stopwatch and a note pad throughout the workday to get the most accurate process steps and times.

As the initial standard work documents are completed, they should be reviewed at two levels: first by all staff members in the clinic who complete that particular task (all nurses, for example, or all physician's assistants) and then by the people who perform the next task in the patient process. This assures the handoffs of information or patient interaction will be smooth. For example, if the physician's assistants are writing standard work for handling x-ray orders, they would logically ask the radiology technologists and the physicians to review the document to ensure that everyone involved knows what information is needed and where that information belongs.

Reviewing and updating standard work documents is a continual process. Each time a new situation, improvement, or problem results in a process change, the standard work must be updated. The standard work document is the definition of the process—as long as those who use it keep it up to date.

Table 6.1 Standard work form.

Title: **Nurse Team Leader Standard Work**
Developed By: **Lori Peterson**
Version: **Final**
Approved By: **Pam Longo**

Step	Activity or Task	Tips for Success (Ideas, Technique, Notes)	Time
1	Before the clinic starts, check patient charts to ensure that the plan, the most recent note, and the flow sheet (if available) are on every chart.	If it seems that the patient might need x-rays, prior to the exam, check in with the doctor or NP.	30 Min
2	During the clinic, if there is a new patient in the exam room, perform an initial assessment to better understand their reason for visiting Orthopedics. Check if x-rays, labs, or other studies have been done.	If the x-rays were not brought along, check with the physician to discuss if he wants x-rays done before seeing the patient.	2 Min/Each
		If CTs, MRIs, or labs were done but not brought along, find out where they were done and call for reports to be faxed to Fax: xxx-xxx-xxxx.	2 Min/Each
3	If there is an FUP patient in the exam room, assess patient status: pain, mobility, ADL isues, school needs, cast/brace issues, emotional concerns and report to MD, Res, or NP prior to the exam.	Report info to MD, Res, or NP.	3-5 Min/Each
4	Work with the Clinic Assistant to monitor wait times, clinic flow, and emergent needs of the patients.	Keep MD, Res, & NP informed of the clinic flow and any immediate patient concerns.	Variable
		Ensure that MD, Res, and NP have clear direction on the next patient to be seen by using the whiteboard.	Variable

WHAT TASKS REQUIRE STANDARD WORK?

For ease of discussion, I'll break the clinic process into two main parts: the time the patient spends with the physician and everything else. The physician's time with the patient is patient-dependent. It's an area where we're keeping our hands off—it is not the first priority for standard work creation. However, everything leading up to the physician's time with the patient and everything after should be standardized—with the goal of setting up the most effective patient-physician interaction possible.

This includes a number of roles and tasks:

Clinic assistant
- How to greet and room patients
- How to question patients and where to write answers on the charts for the PA, resident, or physician
- How to update the whiteboard with patient status

Physician's assistant
- Securing the information the physician wants to know and presenting it as the physician wishes to see it
- How to handle x-ray orders and casting orders
- How to get questions answered regarding casting

Nurse
- What to watch for when the clinic is running behind schedule
- How to set up schedules for the team
- How to perform the team leader role

Physician
- Where to look for information for the next patient
- How to get a debrief before walking into an exam room
- What to write on the whiteboard before and after seeing a patient

Secretaries
- How to work with the systems for scheduling
- How to greet patients
- How to handle late arrivals

Clinic set up

Computers, x-ray PACs systems turned on

Exam room supplies replenished

Cast carts replenished

Whiteboard prepared

Referral forms read

Charts and patient paperwork prepared for next day's clinic

STANDARD WORK IN ACTION

To recap: standard work is a document that defines one person's role in a particular task. It provides a precise description of each work activity, specifying the main process steps. It details, where needed, the time it takes to complete each step and it includes a layout diagram of where each step is completed. Standard work captures the current best way of performing a particular job and gives an organization a method for communicating process improvements systematically to the workforce.

If creating standard work documents sounds like a lot of work, it is. It is a lot of work, it takes a lot of time, and it creates a lot of paperwork. The key is: it's transformational.

"The whole process of standard work, this was extremely enlightening in the early days of implementation," explains Dr. Tassone.

He says candidly: "Most of us didn't really know what everyone else's roles were in clinic. Even more so, we didn't know what everyone thought their roles should be."

In his clinic, the team leaders started the process of drafting standard work documents for nurses and then e-mailed them to the rest of the team for review. One clear benefit, as noted by nurse and team leader Beth Wahlquist, is that "everyone has a voice" in the process and is encouraged to speak up to address concerns or ask questions.

"It was an interesting process," she adds, "because they wouldn't have had the same level of input without Lean. Before the Lean transformation began, tasks were assigned and defined without input from the people actually doing the jobs."

"There was never any discussion around it," she says.

Another visible benefit of creating standard work documents in the Orthopedic Center involved the casting technicians. Some patients need casts and others do not, so the process of assigning times to the cast tech's standard work revealed down time during the course of the workday. With that time identified, cast techs chose to add new skills to their jobs through cross-training and job enrichment. They essentially became resources for other positions in the clinic that experience fluctuating volumes; for example, they could help turn over exam rooms or take on specific administrative tasks during busy times.

And, as nurse Beth Wahlquist notes, "With the standard work documents in place, there's also a very clear way to address deficiencies or issues with work performance. Standard work provides a clear way to say: 'This is how we identified that this job should be done. Why is it not being done that way? How can we fix it?'"

Standard work can result in consistent patient service, no matter what day of the week or who interacts with the patient. Standard work can also reduce patient wait times, especially if each person has analyzed his or her own job, taken the waste out, and created agreed upon best practices.

Ultimately, the focus gets back to patients and their needs, not to broken or inconsistent processes. One of the nurse practitioners in the Orthopedic Center, Allison Duey-Holtz, shares her thoughts on the value of standard work. "We want to ensure the same high quality of care for each patient. The way you become good at something is by repetition. Just as with anything else, practice makes perfect. As you repeat a concept, you also become more efficient at it and the clinic flows even better."

Or as Dr. Tassone explains: "By starting to quantify this and make it concrete, it gave us avenues for improvement. Seeing it also made me more likely to go along with suggested clinic refinements, as I had more insight into why necessary changes were being suggested."

Over time, standard work also becomes the knowledge base for the people using the document. For example, Allison Duey-Holtz (in conjunction with other team members) used the standard work to create best practices for a certain diagnosis of patients that she and her peer physician's assistants and nurse practitioners were beginning to see in increased volumes.

The team reviewed the specific patient population that the group saw in clinic and compared practices. As a joint venture, the physician's assistants and nurse practitioners conducted evidence-based literature searches and agreed on best practices for everyone to follow. For example, now everyone seeing that particular diagnosis asks the patient the same initial questions and knows what answers to expect. She explains that when a patient does not answer as expected or does not fit the profile, the whole team has an opportunity to learn.

Creating standard work for this patient interaction helped assure her that she is providing the best possible care for the patient. "I feel more confident as a provider, that there is less chance of missing things. What we found is that globally everyone was doing similar things with this particular diagnosis, but we each had individual pearls."

These pearls and tips, along with the knowledge from the literature review, helped the team customize and individualize their recommendations to family members, she notes.

"Some people may think that this means we treat each patient as a robot. That is simply not true. We are all humans and adjust to meet the needs of each patient. Having this baseline gives us a great starting point with each patient," she says.

Standard work is commonly used to create flow by creating clear handoffs and responsibilities, and to ensure that each job is properly resourced. This example from Allison Duey-Holtz also shows that standard work can be a great tool to capture medical best practices, especially when evidence-based research and group collaboration through the sharing of experiences provides the foundation.

ACTION STEPS

- Review the standard work template included in the Appendix of this book.

- Identify a starting point for standard work in your practice or clinic. Often, clinic preparation stages, or processes you have changed as a result of your Lean efforts (such as changeover) are good starting points for standard work.

- Ask team members to create a standard work documents for their parts of the process in question, beginning with the work elements and adding details, times, and layouts.

- Conduct reviews of the standard work documents with all those who perform the task and with those who perform the next task in the process.

- Review and update the standard work documents regularly.

7

Step 5 – Lay Out the Clinic for Minimal Motion

This success step is really about the way the physical work environment affects the staff's ability to function as a team. In this chapter, we will dramatically shift our perspective and look at the clinic layout through the staff's eyes—instead of exclusively the patient's eyes—to see where improvements can be made to gain efficiency both in the care process and in team interactions.

To explain this step, I want to note that just about anyone who has ever worked anywhere can share a story about how the work environment affected their performance. My own story comes from early in my career, when I was learning Lean and working in a corporate environment. Each floor of my office building was laid out with offices around the perimeter and elevators in the middle. There were no common areas—no open places where people gathered—just conference rooms and hallways lined with offices. As a result, it was difficult to consult with coworkers or speak face-to-face with stakeholders or others on projects. The communication norm was e-mail, even if the person you were e-mailing was sitting 50 feet down the hallway.

For one project, I worked with an advertising agency located just across the street. It might as well have been a different world. The first time I visited, I was startled at the differences in the layout—and what those differences told me about how work was approached. There were no offices, no hallways, no cubicles. Instead, there were wide open spaces with high counters for impromptu meetings. Open spaces had clusters of arm chairs around coffee tables. Project teams had taken over spaces on the floor, covering the walls with paper for brainstorming sessions. Here, the emphasis was on sharing ideas and getting immediate feedback, on thinking creatively and problem solving. I could tell that much as soon as I walked in.

How people think about their jobs or communicate at work—elements of what is commonly called the work culture—is in part a function of how the workspace is laid out. Of course policies, priorities and management styles also heavily influence culture, but the physical layout plays an important role. If that environment is messy and chaotic, the staff gets the message that operations are also messy and chaotic and without formal processes. If people are separated according to job title—a doctors' work area and a nurses' work area, for example—people get the message that different functions are not expected to communicate. The result is a lost opportunity for richness and synergy that is naturally fostered when workgroups collaborate.

Our goal in this success step is twofold: first, to evaluate the efficiency of your practice's layout and second, to investigate alternatives to the traditional department-based layout that can enhance the flow of communication among the practice's staff. The improvements made to the practice's layout help to further the deep culture changes that move Lean from a quality initiative to an essential part of how your practice and core processes function. When the processes and the physical environment are aligned, the new Lean system quickly becomes "how we do things around here."

So how do we begin?

The main tools we will use for evaluating layout are deceptively simple: 5S and spaghetti diagramming.

DEFINITION OF 5S

5S is the Japanese-developed method for evaluating and improving workplace organization. It evolved as part of Toyota's relentless attempts to remove waste from every process it operates, even at the most detailed level. Imagine a production line worker assembling some small piece of a car. That worker's every move would be observed and analyzed for ways to make it more efficient. The worker is not asked to work faster. Instead, he is asked to simply put the tools he needs closer at hand or to position raw materials in a way that makes them more accessible, so that no motion is wasted. Those small improvements add up to create an environment completely centered on doing value-added work with as little waste as possible. The result is that less time is needed to complete the job, mistakes are harder to make, and ergonomics are improved.

Now imagine the person working at the front desk of your medical practice. Where is the phone? The keyboard? The computer monitor? Where are forms kept? Receipts? How far away are the credit card processor and the patient records? Is that workspace set up for efficiency, based on observation of how the people actually move while doing the job? Are supplies, equipment, and other items in the work area used frequently, or simply stored there because no one knows where else to put them? These are the questions that 5S asks.

One example in a healthcare environment: At my daughters' pediatrician's office, I have to quell the urge to jump over the counter and move the darn printer every time I am there. Instead of acting on this urge, of course, I simply watch in horror as this scene unfolds: first, I pay the office visit co-pay with my debit card; then, the receptionist walks from the counter where I am standing to the back of the office area where a printer generates the credit card form; finally, the receptionist walks to a different area of the counter where the lone stapler is apparently shared among two or three office personnel. Sometimes she is distracted by other demands every step of the way. By the time I sign my name, I have come up with several different layouts for this particularly mundane task. It is a busy office with several doctors; how many times each day does the receptionist walk across the office area? Is that walking value added, or is it waste? It is certainly time-consuming and frustrating for the waiting patient.

How would things change if they asked the questions of 5S? Let's start with a definition. The S's of 5S are translated variously, but we will identify them as Sort, Stabilize, Shine, Standardize, and Sustain. Each is a step of the process. Essentially, the 5S process includes removing everything from the work area that is not used on a daily basis. It can be described as follows:

- **Sort:** separating the necessary from the unnecessary items in the work place and clearing out the clutter.

- **Stabilize:** organizing what's left so that it is readily accessible to the person doing the job.

- **Shine:** cleaning everything to promote pride and attention to the environment.

- **Standardize:** maintaining the changes through formal job responsibilities and policy.

- **Sustain:** This is not exactly a "step" but instead a long-term emphasis on organization and continuous improvement. I'll tackle it in more depth later in this chapter.

The steps are simple and straightforward, yet I am always surprised at what comes out of 5S workshops. One team found a $1 million microscope in a closet filled with cleaning supplies! The microscope had not been used more than once or twice; it had been stored in the closet because no one knew where else to put it. The Lean team checked with the surgeon who ordered it to see whether it could be "red tagged" and removed from the area and whether the surgeon had any plans for it. As it turned out, he had a relationship with a local university and so donated the microscope. The incident made me wonder how many healthcare dollars are tied up in unused equipment hidden away in storage closets.

During a 5S workshop, workers evaluate their own work areas and make changes. Others on the team may help in the evaluation by observing the work in action and sharing those observations, but it is critical that the person doing the job be the one to reorganize the layout of the work area. People take ownership of their desk or work area; it means something to them personally. They may put up pictures, keep snacks in a drawer, and come to think of the workspace as their own, not the organization's. That workspace could be a supply cart, casting room, or cabinet—it doesn't matter. Whatever it is, it is important to someone.

In order to keep that team member engaged in the Lean transformation, you must honor her needs, involve her personally in the 5S work, and keep the focus on the patient. This might seem obvious to you but I had to learn it the hard way, quite painfully, early in my career. I expected that an incoming morning crew of workers would be surprised and delighted by the 5S changes I had led a team to make with the afternoon crew the day before. Well, they were surprised—but delighted is probably not the word they would have used. *Violated*, or *trespassed upon* may have been more accurate! I had to work very hard—and listen to a lot of venting—in order to regain their trust and get their buy-in for the rest of the changes the Lean team wanted to make. Don't make the same mistake.

SPAGHETTI DIAGRAMS

The goal of a 5S workshop is to create the optimal workspace layout for each job in the practice. To do this, the workshop participants observe each job in action and create a spaghetti diagram. A spaghetti diagram is a map that tracks movement in the course of doing a job. To make a spaghetti diagram for nursing, for example, one nurse will observe another with a rough sketch of the room layout in hand. Each time the nurse walks to get something (such as supplies or forms) or otherwise moves, the observer draws a line from the starting point to the ending point. At the end of the observation period, the resulting spaghetti map shows all of the movement: the more movement involved in the job, the more lines on the map (see Figure 7.1).

Once that very visual picture has been created, the goal is to organize the workspace such that the lines on the map are shortened or eliminated altogether. What did that nurse walk away to get? Could that need be filled at the workspace, instead of in a remote supply cabinet or file drawer? What can be taken away (red tagged) from the work area to make room for what's needed?

As the observation goes on, the Lean team members usually begin to ask, "Who designed this place anyway?" The answer is that *no one designed it.* Things are where they are because no one is in charge of keeping the

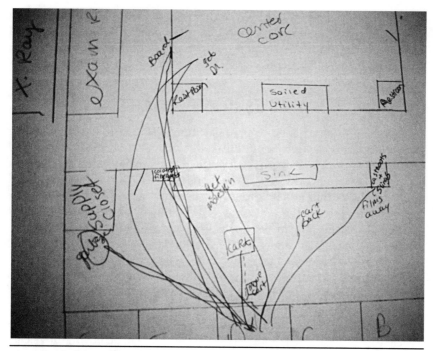

Figure 7.1 Spaghetti diagram.

work area completely focused on efficiency. Forms are hoarded and pile up because once they ran out and that caused a problem. Cabinets contain surprises like $1 million microscopes because cleaning cabinets is tedious and time-consuming and nobody knows where to put abandoned microscopes. Often, how things are stored is a product of years of busy operation without the chance to step back and analyze the system.

Once the spaghetti maps are created, the team uses its knowledge of Lean principles to organize the workstations, clear out the clutter, and make sure the necessary supplies are exactly where they are needed. The team can conduct quick experiments with the layout by performing the job and getting immediate feedback about placement of equipment and supplies. Ultimately, the workspace organization should promote efficiency in the job, as well as healthy ergonomics and a focus on the relentless improvement of the care processes.

There are many good examples of 5S in clinics. Commonly used forms (such as excuse or education) can be placed in the exam rooms for convenient staff access. Commonly needed supplies (Band-Aids, tape, suture removal kits, and so on) can be placed in exam rooms or close by in a conveniently located supply cart. At check-in stage for the patients, the secretary's work can be analyzed to place commonly used forms (and printers!) close at hand. Once during a 5S event in the Emergency Department, we cleared a cluttered exam room that was never used because it was full of forms and equipment. You never know what you may find during a 5S event.

WHY 5S IS IMPORTANT

Without 5S, other changes are much more difficult to make. Working in a place that pays no attention to the organization of its forms and tools and supplies is like asking a distractible child to sit at a messy desk to do homework—the distractions and the clutter take over and make the work that much harder to do. 5S and its attention to the work environment creates the atmosphere that allows other, more significant changes to occur. 5S can also help improve patient satisfaction scores, because patients may feel a sense of control and well-being while visiting your clean and organized facility.

Done well, 5S supports all of the other success steps laid out in this book. Remember when we talked about physician flow in Chapter 3 and I described the need to treat all of the steps in the care process (other than face-to-face time with the patient) as turnover, and to do them as efficiently as possible? I compared the staff's role in achieving physician flow to that of a pit crew, working as one unit on a shared goal. But the pit crew would not be effective if one of its members had to run back to the office for a wrench, or if the gas pump was located too far away to reach the car. And remember the role of team leaders, discussed in Chapter 4? Well, they need an organized work environment that places emphasis on process excellence in order to orchestrate the activity of the staff and maintain the Lean system. And visual communication (Chapter 5) provides clear information and real-time decision making, but only if the message is visible and not lost in a cluttered work environment! All of the changes we've made until this point will be supported and enhanced by 5S.

PULL SYSTEMS AND SUPERMARKETS FOR SUPPLIES REPLENISHMENT

When the supplies, materials and equipment are organized and placed in such a way that the worker does not waste motion in the course of the job, the next logical step is to look at how those supplies get replenished. The practice will not be able to sustain the system of organization if supplies run out (causing people to hoard secret stashes) or if suppliers deliver inappropriate quantities of forms or supplies that have to be stored in hallways or clutter up cabinets.

The last of the 5S's—Sustain—involves creating a system to ensure that the work done during a 5S workshop is not lost. A good, thorough cleaning can be motivating for the team, but the work environment will not stay that way on its own. It will need continual maintenance. To maintain the organization and orderliness of supplies and forms, we apply the concept of material pull. Pull is established using a kanban card system or by creating a supermarket for high-volume forms and supplies. When the inventory of supplies in the supermarket reaches a predetermined minimum quantity (based on the amount of time it takes to replenish the material) the clinic orders more. (See Figure 7.2.)

Pull System
A system in which no material or product moves until the next process is ready for it.

Supermarket
A controlled inventory of needed materials or supplies. In the clinic, a supermarket could be a quantity of forms or a cart of casting supplies.

Kanban
A card that accompanies materials. When the material is to be reordered, the card is sent back to the supplying process to trigger a delivery to the supermarket.

For example, intake paperwork forms are common at the front desks of medical practices, and are used in high volume. As such, they are good candidates for management through a supermarket. If the receptionist uses 20 forms per day and the internal supplier can deliver more forms with a half-day's notice, then a replenishment order would be placed when the forms get down to 10. The clinic would only order the number of forms it can store without taking up space designated for other materials. This system would prevent the receptionist from running out of forms, and would also prevent the internal supplier from delivering so many that they become clutter.

Material pull in the practice helps to maintain an orderly environment because what's on hand is only what is needed. Further, establishing pull with internal suppliers means driving your Lean initiative across departmental boundaries, thus clarifying requirements and reducing the possibility for errors caused by supplying functions.

Depending on the lead time of external suppliers, it may make sense to have a central materials supermarket in the practice. This intermediate step would reduce space requirements for forms storage. If external

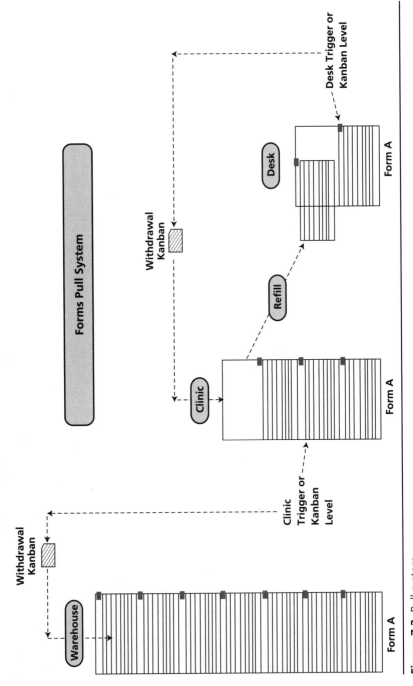

Figure 7.2 Pull system.

suppliers can deliver more materials quickly, this intermediate step can be eliminated. But if the lead time is too long, a supermarket provides a "buffer" inventory to help make sure the practice does not run out of a critical material.

LAYOUT CONSIDERATIONS FOR THE ENTIRE PRACTICE

Mapping and improving individual workspaces is just one part of a thorough 5S application. Those workspaces are all part of a larger whole: it is important to see how people and information move through them from wall to wall in the practice. In keeping with that value stream approach, the next level of 5S for the practice uses spaghetti maps to illustrate the communication and movement of all team members in the process of patient care.

Individual spaghetti mapping asked the question, "Where should supplies and equipment be located to help this person do her job most efficiently?" In contrast, spaghetti mapping for the entire practice asks questions such as, "How many times did the physician go to someone else to ask a question?" "Where are supporting departments such as radiology or physical therapy?" "Where are the break room and the coffee machine?" "How far are the nurses from the rest of the team?" "How much information is passed along verbally in the hallways?"

The map captures interactions among staff members to highlight where questions, clarifications, or instructions add to patient wait times as physicians, nurses, and other staff cross and re-cross the clinic for needed information.

Once the map reveals the extent to which the team is dependent upon each other for information, the physical barriers to effective communication become clear. These barriers include long hallways of exam rooms that prevent staff from seeing each other or the patient status board; supporting departments that are located at the far end of the clinic and isolate staff members who need to interface with the clinic staff; and workstations set up by job title that prevent the staff of the clinic from acting like a coordinated team. Even a break room designed to keep coffee-drinking staff out of the view of patients adds to the staff's difficulty in finding people and information in the moment they are needed.

Creating spaghetti maps at this level highlights changes that can positively impact patient wait times. Often we find the proverbial low-hanging fruit—file cabinets in the wrong locations, shared supplies that could be distributed differently, or information that could be added to the patient status board. Sometimes the implications are less obvious—work areas that isolate some staff members, information that is chronically missing and must be tracked down, or weak information handoffs between functions. Once the team sees the results of these issues on movement through the clinic, solutions can be readily generated.

PRECONSTRUCTION CONSIDERATIONS

All of the steps described here can help an existing clinic or practice use its space more efficiently, but we also want to take this exercise a step further. Consider the possibilities available if you're building a new clinic or an addition to an existing clinic, or even constructing a shell space within an existing building or remodeling an existing site. This provides a great opportunity to rethink traditional layouts and design facilities for minimal patient and staff motion. When minimal patient wait times are the primary design consideration, clinic planners must ask themselves a new set of questions to break through old paradigms about what a clinic should look like:

- Should supporting departments have doors that open to a common workroom so the staff can easily access the physician (and vice versa)?
- Rather than a nursing station, should there instead be a team station to remove the physical barriers to communication?
- Should exam rooms be arranged in a semi-circle so the physician has visual communication with the staff no matter what room he's in?
- Would a high, communal work counter promote teamwork better than individual desks or offices?
- Are the exam rooms designed around the patient assessment process?
- Are exam room cabinets big enough for storage of supplies at the point of use?

Children's Hospital of Wisconsin had such an opportunity to ask those questions in 2007 when it designed its Greenway clinics building, a remote site. Orthopedics was one of the specialties that would be setting up operations at Greenway, and so Terry Schwartz, the Orthopedics program administrator, was involved in the final stage of the design process. The story of her involvement in the Greenway clinic design is one of extraordinary foresight.

Shortly before the Orthopedic Center space was finalized, she was given two plans from the hospital's architects and asked to choose between plan A and plan B. Knowing what she did about patient and physician flow, as well as about the overall patient experience, she did not like either plan. She asked for time to come up with plan C and was given two weeks. In those two weeks, she talked to the critical stakeholders, consulted with me, and sketched out a floor plan that reflected everything she had come to learn about process flow and communication.

Her new plan had three critical elements: an extra door to each exam room; a common work area for all the clinic staff, including the physicians; and a co-located radiology department. (See Figure 7.3.) She had to fight for the extra door, she explains, because of the added cost. But the benefits are invaluable. When patients are shown to an exam room, they walk along an exterior wall lined with windows. They enter an exam room from that hallway and never see the staff work area or any of the "behind the scenes" workings of the clinic. It's a remarkable experience for the patients and their families, as the experience is much more peaceful and organized. The staff enters the same exam room from the second door, which leads to the common workroom. (This setup is sometimes known as "on stage" and "off stage;" Dr. Tassone had been familiar with it from his work in another clinic.) So while the staff is in constant communication with each other and has access to the patient status board, files, supplies, and computers, the patient sees nothing but a nice view out the windows and the exam room.

Quiet, Stress-Free Visit

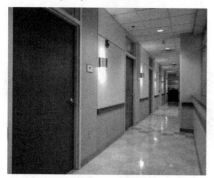

Multi-Function Cast/Exam Rooms

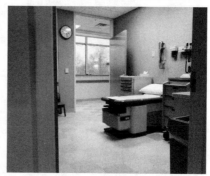

On-Stage/Off-Stage

Figure 7.3 Two-door room layout.

Privacy is another benefit of the second door. Because the second door faces the staff work area, patients' charts can be hung on the door without being visible to other patients walking by. In other clinics, patient charts have to be placed face down on the door to protect privacy so that sensitive information is not displayed to all those walking through common hallways.

The common workroom also does several things at once (see Figure 7.4). Practically, it provides an area to sit down and work. Doctors and residents do their dictating at a high counter that is conducive to working while standing, and thereby makes the most use of the five-minute or ten-minute slots of available time to which the team leader will alert the physician. Computers on the counter are used for looking up information for patients while those patients are still in the exam rooms. From a team perspective, the common workroom erases the boundaries between job titles. Nurses, cast techs, nurse practitioners, physician's assistants, and physicians all share a space. All exam rooms open into the common work area, so when a provider has a question or needs assistance, help can be found easily. Just as important, that common space fosters an environment in which all voices are heard equally, in which the nurse or the cast tech can challenge the physician, for example, or in which the team leader can maintain a focus on the process.

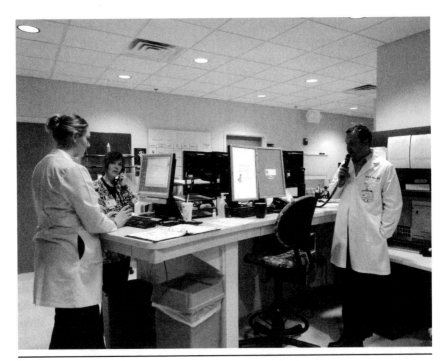

Figure 7.4 Common work area.

It is important to note that the idea of a common workroom only works when that workroom is devoted to one physician's team. When the workroom houses staff from more than one practice, the resulting noise and distractions defeat the purpose of having the physician and her staff close together. It is no easier to find the right person or information in a crowd than it is in a long and deserted hallway. The goal is to create a team space for each physician practice to enable productive communication and the sharing of ideas and information. It doesn't work to segregate the team by job title in separate rooms, nor does it work to create one big space for all the practices in the clinic or hospital.

Placing Radiology in the Orthopedic Center space simplifies the process for patients and ensures that they do not get "lost" when they need to have an x-ray as part of the visit. Over time, several benefits have emerged from the decision to integrate Radiology in the new center. First, the patient is occasionally able to go directly to Radiology to have a cast removed by a cast technician before he is put into an exam room. That eliminates the wait in the exam room and makes full use of the clinic's mobile casting carts.

Second, being co-located with the Orthopedics staff has made it much easier for the radiology technologists to have questions answered in real time. In the past, finding the right people to answer questions about Radiology orders was too difficult and took too much time, leaving the technologists in the difficult position of having to interpret orders or use their past experience to take an educated guess as to what is needed. If they did not interpret the orders correctly, further delays ensued because the films had to be done again. Now, the Radiology staff can see the Orthopedic workroom from where they are located and can easily find the physician to ask for clarification without causing delays or backups at their own function.

Finally, the Radiology technologists are able to specialize and gain a deeper expertise in the arena of Orthopedics, thus becoming more valuable resources to the organization and its patients.

Again, these types of questions can work and these improvements can be made whether you're building an entirely new site or working within the confines of redesign.

WHAT TO DO WHEN YOU CANNOT BUILD NEW WALLS

Whenever we talk about layout changes with our clients, their first response is to go looking for a sledgehammer. "If only we could tear down that wall!" they all seem to say—and they are right. Tearing down walls—or building new ones—is an appealing option for achieving flow. Once the team learns to see the process from the value stream perspective and experience it as the patient does, the realization that the physical building was not created with flow in mind is never far behind.

Unfortunately, though, few organizations are willing or able to undertake major renovations as part of their Lean transformation—at least not as an early step. So what do you do when you literally hit that brick wall?

Significant changes can be made to existing practices to improve communication flow and reduce patient wait times. Perhaps nothing can be done about that long hallway of exam rooms, but how the exam rooms and workstations are used can be rethought. First, remember that the goal is to create a team space, not necessarily a Greenway-style common workroom. Common workrooms are great, but they are simply a way to achieve a greater sense of teamwork and collaboration.

We have found an effective alternative method for achieving that sense of teamwork when the dedicated physical space is simply not available. The first step is to have the practice nurse begin to act like the team leader. She should work the same days as the physician for consistency and begin to take ownership for supporting the physician's value-added time.

Next, look carefully at the work processes in the practice and define the role that each person plays. Role confusion causes many misunderstandings and dropped balls in patient care; in order to function and collaborate like a team, everyone in the practice must understand clearly what is expected of them. (For more on this, see the chapter on standard work.)

Then make a space for the nurse to sit next to the physician, and make sure there is a computer there. This sounds like a simple step, and indeed it is. But the simple act of putting the nurse and physician next to each other will facilitate the nurse's role of team leader and help the physician stay in contact. The nurse can update the patient status board and alert the physician to scheduling issues or available time. They can work in tandem to ensure that patients flow through the practice.

One organization we worked with had a newly built nurses' room in a large clinic care practice. In this practice, the nurses were already paired with physicians with whom they worked consistently. Those nurses almost immediately abandoned the new nurses' room and moved their computers next to the physicians because most of that they do is in contact with that physician. Separating them by job title just didn't make sense.

Not just the nurse/team leader but the physician's entire core team should sit as close to each other as possible given the space you have. If your space is too small to bring the entire team together, then the first priority is to bring the physician and the nurse/team leader together. The rest of the team—the nurse practitioner, the physician's assistant and others—should sit as close to each other as they can as well, but the space can be separated from the physician and team leader. When that small group space is designated, create a glass wall for the team and put it up right next to where the team sits.

The final step is to make any services portable that can be, such as forms and supplies, so that the team leader need not leave the common area to perform her job. When the team leader has everything she needs in the common area, the work is focused more clearly on the patient-physician interaction.

ACTION STEPS

- Create spaghetti diagrams of work areas to be improved.

- Conduct a 5S workshop to redesign the work area. Clear out clutter and unnecessary materials and organize what is left to improve the layout and reduce the number of lines on the spaghetti diagram.

- Determine whether a supermarket and pull system is appropriate for high-volume forms and supplies.

- Investigate alternatives for creating a common workspace for the practice team to facilitate the flow of communication.

8
Step 6 – Change the Care Delivery Model

A nd so, at this last step along our Lean journey, we return to our starting point: creating processes that truly put patients at the center of the healthcare environment.

Wait a minute! Haven't we done that already?

Yes, but not quite. It turns out that the first five success steps are foundation steps—they make changes that indeed are important in themselves and they make changes that allow real innovations to occur. This is because the process has to be as stable and as free of waste and confusion as possible before any big, paradigm-shifting changes can occur.

Think of it like this: when you hear about radically different models of care delivery—such as a kiosk in the Emergency Department for children with ear infections—it is safe to assume that the big change (the kiosk) is the tip of the iceberg. What is not so visible is the system underneath that allowed the change to be possible.

To better explain, I'll tell you about the an exercise we often use to start Lean training sessions. For it, we place the participants in a large circle and ask them to throw tennis balls to each other in a particular order. We call this their "process," and we time it to see how long it takes them to throw and catch the balls. We then ask them to operate that process— throw and catch the tennis balls—faster and faster without dropping the balls. The pressure to catch the balls and throw them quickly causes stress and problems and the time it takes for the team to complete its "process" goes up. Eventually, we let them confer with each other about how to redesign the process by standing closer to each other or handing the balls to each other instead of throwing them, and their times go from a minute or more to perhaps 10 seconds. Once they reach that point, we tell them that the benchmark, best-in-class tennis ball time is 0.5 seconds. Invariably, they are inspired to be creative and hit that benchmark.

I know from experience that they would not succeed in achieving that time if I told them the benchmark while they were still throwing (and dropping) the balls and taking a minute to do so. It's only after they have removed some of the confusion and waste from their original process that they are ready to take on what would have seemed like an impossible challenge.

The same is true for a Lean transformation.

People who cannot find the right equipment to do their jobs, or who are still hoarding supplies because of inventory problems, or who cannot talk directly to the physician they are supporting because of personality issues are not remotely ready to think about drive-through emergency department services. Basic process stability must be achieved first. Once it has been achieved, though, the next steps are just about as wide open as the big blue sky.

OLD SYSTEMS, NEW SYSTEMS, BORROWED SYSTEMS

So what does changing the care delivery model mean? It means exactly what we've been discussing all along: re-imagining the care process and changing the paradigm to make it patient centered. Often, the old systems originated for the ease of the physician because the physician's time is limited and valuable and patients are plentiful.

It made sense for the physician to line up lots of patients in the casting area, for example, see them quickly, write the orders for casts, and move on. Meanwhile, exam rooms fill up and the physician has another batch of patients waiting. That physician wastes little time, but what about the patients? (Remember how Children's Marketing Director Julie Pedretti described this: "Our systems have always been around the providers, what is convenient for the physician. How does it work for our medical staff model? How does it fit in with our clinical appointment scheduling system? That's not about the patient.")

And so the question: What about the patient? That is at the heart of this most transformative success step.

The success steps you've completed so far help you achieve process stability—which is required before it's possible to take the next big step and change the paradigm of how care is delivered. And that's our final success step—to make care delivery truly patient centered and eliminate the queues that create that false efficiency for the doctor.

A LOOK BACK AT CHANGING THE MODEL IN MANUFACTURING

Manufacturing is a good place to look to observe the changing model from departments to cells. Traditional manufacturing is made up of departments. In my early career as a process engineer, I worked for a coatings manufacturer that organized its plants into departments. Each department completed one particular part of the manufacturing process: preassembling raw materials, mixing the coatings, testing the coatings, filling the coatings into shipping containers, and shipping them from the warehouse. Between the departments, the product moved around the factory on fork trucks and was stored on racks or on the factory floor. Each department was managed separately with its own supervisor, its own schedule, and its own goals for production and efficiency.

The problems with this model are obvious in retrospect: Moving material around is a non-value added task that takes up time, costs money, and potentially results in damage and loss of materials. Individual department schedules are difficult to coordinate over an entire manufacturing operation and result in a "feast or famine" production environment in which some functions are overloaded and others have nothing to do. Overproduced material sits in aisles and warehouses, sometimes for so long that the product becomes obsolete and becomes another cost to the company.

By contrast, Lean creates small "mini-factories" or *cells* that produce one type of product in one area that contains all of the equipment necessary for that product. The equipment is arranged so that the product travels the shortest distance from the beginning to the end of the manufacturing process. By aligning resources and equipment around the product (rather than making the product travel to the resources and equipment) much of the waste and non-value added activity is removed from the manufacturing process. There is no need for legions of fork trucks to transport material from one place to another, and one schedule controls the work for the entire cell. The operation becomes much simpler, allowing for higher quality and greater efficiency.

CELLS IN THE HEALTHCARE SETTING

Healthcare organizations are often organized in departments that resemble traditional manufacturing. (See Figure 8.1.) There is a high need for transportation among departments, and scheduling is complex. But if we align resources and equipment around the patient (rather than making the patient travel to the resources and equipment), we can create a truly patient-centered organization. The first and most obvious way to do this is through the creation of cells. A cell eliminates many different sources of waste—the motion of walking (or driving) from one provider area to another, the over-processing of duplicated data gathering, and even potential defects caused by redundant care or poor communication among functions or organizations.

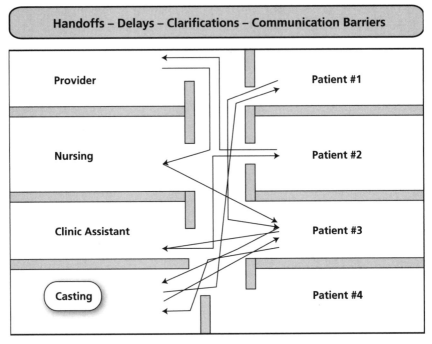

Figure 8.1 Traditional departmental layout.

A cell that is functioning well has a beautiful simplicity to it. From the patient's point of view, no paradigm has been changed at all, the care process has simply been made more convenient and more understandable. (See Figure 8.2.)

In order to create a functioning cell, the first step is to evaluate the types of patients coming to your practice. Even within specialties, there are "patient families," groups of patients who have similar needs and require similar services. In orthopedics, for example, patient families are easy to see and differentiate. A fracture patient is much different than a scoliosis patient; a sports injury or head injury may require different support services than a baby born with a club foot. Each of these examples belongs in a different patient family, and each patient family should ideally be treated in its own cell.

To analyze your patient families, create a matrix that lists all of the possible supporting functions with which your patients interface and the categories of patients that you see. Wherever the majority of steps in the process are the same for a patient category, you have a patient family around which the cell can be created. You may find that you send 20 percent of your patients for certain lab tests or diagnostic imaging; that volume may be enough to build the business case for bringing that lab or imaging service into the practice and creating a cell.

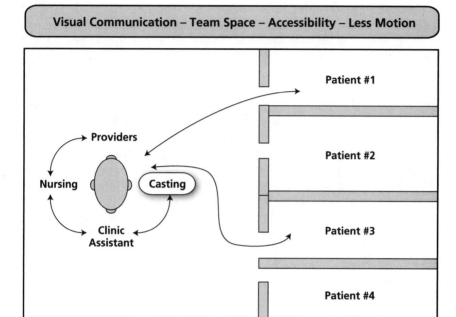

In this illustration, a common staff area facilitates better communication and easier access to staff members.

Figure 8.2 Cell layout.

Once the patient families have been identified, the next step is to schedule them separately. Creating a cell does not mean building a new facility for each patient family; rather, it means scheduling them separately so that a scoliosis patient who needs 30 minutes of the physician's time is not causing three or four 10-minute fracture patients to wait. Many clinics have already taken this step outside of a Lean effort in order to simplify scheduling and avoid chaos. Each patient family is a separate clinic, scheduled on a particular day or time period: fractures on Monday afternoons and Wednesday mornings, sports injuries on Tuesdays, spine patients on Fridays.

The cell, then, is the patient family being serviced by the physician and the physician's team using the tools and philosophies described in the first five success steps. Ideally, within this cell the services should travel to the patient in the exam room. This is where mobile supply carts and services such as mobile cast carts come into play. Now, rather than being a misapplied part of a wide Lean effort, those mobile carts are supporting a thoughtfully planned and thoroughly supported Lean system.

Providing services in the exam room is the easiest cell-creation step to execute. Next in difficulty and expense is relocating supporting functions to be in the same physical space as the physician practice. In one patient family, the common step may be a test conducted in the lab or a need for a trip to the pharmacy. Including that care step in the cell would mean creating the ability to conduct the test in the practice or locating a pharmacy in the same space. In both of these examples, the requirement is to be able to service the product family, not build a fully-stocked pharmacy or a lab capable of servicing the entire organization. The cell provides specific services to a specific group of patients.

Outside the physician practice, the cell takes on a wider application. Healthcare organizations have created large cells that provide many services to a broad patient family—women's care centers, for example, or heart centers. These cells typically have many physicians and provide care for a broad range of patient families within a specialty. The best of these have the ability to provide supporting functions under the same roof (ultrasound capability, for example, in a women's care center) so that patients with complex needs experience coordinated care.

NEXT STEPS IN CARE DELIVERY

A cell functions well when the right patients are being cared for by physicians who are focused on the patient/physician consultation and supported by a team that knows what to do when and has patient satisfaction as its common goal. At the beginning of this book, we said that when patients are flowing through the practice, a great many things are going right. The functioning cell is the culmination of all of those things.

When the cell is functioning smoothly, the physician and the practice managers are free to look up from the clinic activity and investigate other options for care—that's where the innovative, ground-breaking ideas come from. These could include that drive-through lane in the ER for ear infections, innovative preventive measures in the community, or the inclusion of alternative care such as acupuncture. What they are specifically really isn't the point. The point is that they cannot be achieved—or even conceptualized—until the foundation of process stability, patient focus, and standardization is laid.

THIS STEP IN ACTION AT
THE ORTHOPEDIC CENTER

Remember: With this final step, changing the care delivery model means being able to put ourselves in the shoes of the patient from both a convenience standpoint and a medical standpoint. For convenience, it comes down to motion of the patients—whether they are walking around from department to department or making multiple trips to the hospital for labs, radiology, echo, and so on. From a Lean standpoint, the equation is this: How much time is spent receiving medical services and how much time is spent waiting or walking around?

When we look at things medically, this convenience also has better care written all over it. For example, one small change we made at the Orthopedic Center at Children's actually shifted the entire paradigm of how care was delivered. The change seems simple in hindsight: Rather than having a patient leave the exam room and move to a casting room, where the casting technicians would put on the cast, we moved the casting technicians to the exam room.

The benefits: The patient does not have to move and the casting technician is now located close to the physician. This can be especially important when, as Dr. Tassone notes, he is not sure of the feasibility of a specific cast in a given situation. The new arrangement allows the cast tech and Dr. Tassone to come up with a solution on the spot.

When we proposed this change, it met with great skepticism and resistance. As Dr. Tassone notes: "I was greatly skeptical at first. It just wasn't the way I did it. But I was willing to give it a try, and now I can't imagine it any other way."

The fundamental lesson: Having processes physically apart leads to poor communication, faulty assumptions, and perhaps not the best care for the patient.

We also saw evidence of this when we moved Radiology to shared space in the Greenway clinic described in the previous chapter. (See Figure 8.3.) In the previous arrangement, with Radiology located physically apart from Orthopedics, the radiology technician might have taken the wrong x-ray, if the instructions weren't perfectly clear, and sent the patient back to the clinic. Eventually the patient would be sent back to Radiology for the correct x-ray. At Greenway, the radiology technologists are now able to talk to the physician without having the patient move from the radiology table. This not only means less wait time, it means fewer errors, fewer x-rays, and less radiation for the patients.

Now let's imagine more possibilities. For example, Dr. Tassone notes that the specialist known as the orthotist—who measures and makes customized braces for spine patients—is located somewhere else in the hospital. Wouldn't it be great if that specialty were co-located with the Orthopedic department so that the patient would get the right brace quickly, rather than having to walk around the hospital? This isn't just about wasted steps. As Dr. Tassone notes, it's also about medical communication between the physician and the orthotist, about being able to ask "What if?" and engage in joint decision-making that would ultimately lead to a better brace solution for the patient. Just like our cast tech or radiology technician, the orthotist would have access to Dr. Tassone for specific questions and details.

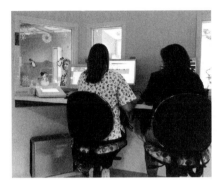

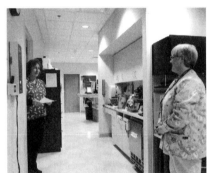

Figure 8.3 Radiology integrated within clinic.

I want to note that there are clear business-based reasons to rethink these processes—for instance, Children's Hospital of Wisconsin is based in Milwaukee but strives to target patients from throughout the Midwest. They won't be able to attract these patients for long if patients who are willing to take the long drive then have to wait long times for their appointments or have bad experiences with care. As Julie Pedretti noted, bad word of mouth and bad perceptions are very costly to change. And yes, we addressed this with the first five success steps.

But now you can take it one step further. Imagine a system that was truly centered on the sick child, the child who needs care. Most children being seen regularly at a pediatric hospital have a range of related medical problems. Let's listen to what Julie has to say about serving them, and imagine the possibilities:

"We've got good market share in Milwaukee. Our interest is expanding geographically more of the Midwest market, which is our primary market. We do want to provide the best care for pediatrics, especially with certain types of diagnosis here.

"What Lean allows us to do as a system or tool—especially with those complicated cases with kids who need to see multiple providers—is to think about developing a system that allows us to schedule all of their care during the stay, whether it's a day or two or a week. Not when it's convenient to the providers, when they have openings, but a system that allows us to schedule around the child. That is key. It is more than concierge services, it's being able to provide access to the right physicians and care at the right time. It can't be silos. It has to be an integrated system."

Your Lean transformation allows you to think about things like this, to reconsider the possibilities, to make your healthcare setting truly patient centered. Lean allows you to create a vision. Without a vision, everything is impossible. With a vision, well, you can imagine and create the possibilities, one success step at a time.

ACTION STEPS

- Analyze the patients seen in your practice or clinic to determine patient families. Use a matrix listing the supporting functions or other high-volume steps to facilitate this analysis.

- Based on your patient family analysis, build a business case for bringing supporting functions into the practice and creating a cell.

- Schedule patient families (cells) separately.

- Bring services to patients in the exam rooms to eliminate patient travel within the cell.

- Spend some time imagining "What if" scenarios beyond the walls of your practice to create patient flow and improve care.

Lean Leadership

Focus on wait times. Start with the physician. Implement the success steps. Poof! Your healthcare organization will magically transform and everything will be better, right?

Not so fast. The philosophies and tools we've presented so far work and will yield results, but there is another part of the picture that we have only partly addressed: you. Since you're reading this book, you presumably have an interest in Lean and what it can do for your healthcare organization. You play a big role in whether Lean can transform your practice or clinic or hospital as powerfully as it did the Orthopedic Center at Children's Hospital. In order for you to play that role effectively, you must understand some things about Lean leadership.

As you've surely noticed me repeating throughout this book, Lean is a philosophy that is "pulled" from the bottom up rather than "pushed" from the top down. This is so vital to the success of a Lean transformation. It must be "owned" by the front line workers in any organization, the people who do the nitty-gritty day-to-day detail work. And yet, here is the paradox: Making an effort like this truly successful and truly transformative involves a tremendous amount of leadership.

Before going into more detail about this, I want some of the leaders at Children's to address their ideas of leadership and what leadership qualities made the Orthopedic Center transformation so successful.

First, chief quality officer and corporate vice president Dr. Ramesh Sachdeva notes that a successful Lean transformation "requires resources and commitment from senior leadership. It is not something that you just do on a weekend. It requires commitment. In our case, we had a complete commitment from our Executive Vice President, Cindy Christensen. Very candidly, if she had not been committed to that extent, I do not know if we could have been that successful."

Commitment from senior leadership indeed is key. Later in this chapter, we will touch on ways that Lean leaders can communicate important details about their Lean transformation to key executives, opening doors with the organization's most senior leaders.

Next, from hospital vice president Lee Ann Eddy, who oversaw the Orthopedic department: "Finding the right manager for the process was key—who was the correct leader to begin this journey? I knew we needed someone who was willing to make the commitment, someone who would be able to lead her team."

If you're the manager overseeing a Lean transformation, we'll offer suggestions for appropriate ways to lead and manage your team.

Finally, Orthopedic surgeon Dr. Channing Tassone, who was our physician champion and leader on so many levels of the transformation, gives a perspective on leadership in the healthcare environment that is remarkably insightful and one that's rarely discussed when talking about physicians.

He notes: "All physicians think that they are 'a leader' and the leader of their practice. While on some level this is true, this experience with Lean has helped me to realize that while we may be leading, we aren't leading in a cohesive and structured fashion. We are simply doing what we think works best, usually based solely on anecdotal experience that we observed during our medical training. We assume that the way we saw 'successful' clinics run must be the best way to do things. Working with Lean has forced me to take a step back and re-evaluate my 'leadership,' if it really even should be called that."

The physician champion involved with the Lean transformation plays a vital leadership role in its success. In fact, physicians play a most important leadership role in any healthcare setting. And yet it's interesting to note how little training physicians actually receive about business leadership principles—even though they lead their clinics or practices every day.

Dr. Tassone says: "What we call leadership is really just us showing up for work and trying to get the work done. This may work in the most basic of practices—but even in those, *true leadership* has an opportunity to vastly improve patient care, personal satisfaction of the provider, and team satisfaction of all of the colleagues that we are working with."

He adds: "This has also made me realize that leadership styles may need to adapt over time, and in different environments. The clinic, the operating room, the emergency department, and one's office may and likely do require variations on one's leadership style and utilizing different skills."

Developing leadership skills is clearly a vital step to making the Lean transformation successful.

And so I'll say that the goal of Lean leadership is to engage the hearts and minds of the people involved in every step of the care delivery process. They must feel ownership for the whole system, not just their part of it, in order to imagine solutions that will transform care. They must build a sense of community in the clinic or hospital or practice so that solutions and changes can be presented without the blame and defensiveness that so often go along with improvement efforts. Finally, they must all speak the same language so that they can erase the barriers of education and rank that separate medical professionals and keep opinions from being offered equally.

These three elements—ownership for the whole system, a sense of community, and a common language—must be intentionally built by a person leading the Lean transformation: by you. Maybe you are the doctor who feels called to manage your practice differently. Maybe you are the clinic manager or an executive who envisions a more efficient and effective future with Lean. Maybe you are a change agent without any positional authority who is interested in what Lean can do for the organization. No matter what your role, the leadership competencies we will discuss in this chapter apply to you just as much as the six success steps do.

There is, of course, a lot of literature already written about the qualities of business leadership. I'm devoting time to it here because I have found that the leadership style of the person driving the Lean transformation profoundly impacts whether Lean changes will be lasting and sustainable. And I will devote time to it here because leading a Lean transformation does truly run counter to the traditional view of management: It's not the leader who delegates the most or drives the toughest bargain or manages the numbers the closest who is successful with Lean. To create a new system, you must use a new set of skills.

> Director of Quality Data Management (QDM) Stephanie Lenzner describes an underlying assumption, that doctors went into medicine because they want to help and heal (among other motivators). And so a value proposition such as "Improve the patient experience" can be vaguely insulting to a doctor—implying they're not already doing everything they can. They are trained to diagnose, to figure out what is wrong. Their minds are already there. Instead, benefits must be personalized under the assumption that helping the patient is already a motivator.

LEADERSHIP COMPETENCY MODEL

A competency model is a list of skills, traits, and behaviors that describe what is needed to do a particular job well. This competency model for Lean leaders was developed with input from people who had successfully led a Lean initiative in our client organizations and with the observations of our consultants. (See Figure III.1.)

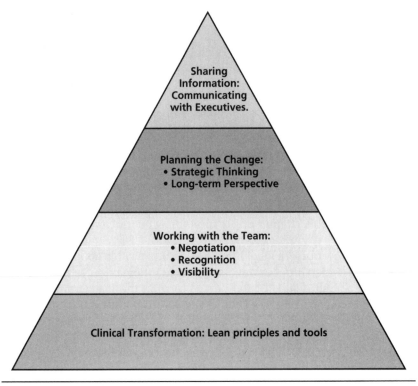

Figure III.1 Lean leader competency model.

At the base of the model are the tools and principles of clinical transformation that are described in the rest of this workbook. Without a strong foundation in Lean and the methodology needed to apply it to the clinic setting, leading this kind of Lean effort would be impossible.

The next tier describes competencies needed for creating change within a group of people. These are the critical interpersonal skills: negotiation as a conflict reducing measure, visibility and leading by example, and providing feedback to the team.

Next on the model are the competencies needed to plan a logical progression of changes to transform the clinic. Lean leaders must think two or three steps down the road as they plan changes and workshops. Often, one workshop lays the foundation for a change that will take place a few months later; therefore, the plan must extend beyond simply the next event. Developing that kind of strategic thinking means looking at your Lean activities with a long-term perspective and realizing that sustainable change does not occur on a short timeline.

The top of the pyramid is communicating with executives. This may be a competency you use infrequently; however, it is vital to your ability to remove major roadblocks in the implementation (and perhaps vital to your career as well). No major change takes place in a vacuum. You must keep sponsors and champions up to date on your progress and challenges by communicating effectively through the management structures of your organization.

WORKING WITH THE TEAM

Negotiation

Negotiation is a basic tool for getting what you want from others, a way to reach an agreement when you and the other side have some interests in common and some that are opposed. We negotiate all the time, deciding what to do on a Saturday evening, who will do the dishes, how we'll communicate patient status in the clinic, and what elements will be included in standard work.

Negotiation is a more useful competency for a Lean leader than conflict management, even though the two are closely related. Conflict, in a change scenario, is the result of failed negotiations. My favorite example of this comes not from my consulting work, but from my home life. My wife, Carolyn, and I attended the same Lean Manufacturing training soon after we were married. In my enthusiasm to implement what I had learned, I reorganized our kitchen and pantry while she was not at home. I zealously applied 5S to the pantry shelves, labeling bins for different food types and setting reorder points. In the kitchen I moved small appliances around to better position them for their purpose, and put the coffee maker near the refrigerator where the cream was kept.

I forgot, though, that my wife is the front-line operator in that kitchen and she drinks her coffee black. When she came home and saw the results of my kitchen 5S workshop, she went through the roof—just as (she tells me) any reasonable person would when his or her workspace is rearranged without permission or input. Had I viewed this as an opportunity for negotiation and not just jumped into the changes I thought were necessary, I could have avoided a lot of conflict.

In their classic book, *Getting to Yes*, William Ury and Roger Fisher advocate moving away from positions in negotiations and focusing on interests. A position is an unequivocal statement ("I want the whiteboard hung here") that backs the negotiator into a corner and generates conflict. An interest ("I want the whiteboard to be highly visible") allows the people in the negotiation to generate several alternative solutions and find one that is satisfactory to all.

There are many negotiations—big and small—that take place during a Lean transformation. You must negotiate to get small changes trialed, to secure the team's energy and attention during a busy day, and to gain access to resources in other departments. The key to being able to focus on interests, rather than positions, is the data collection a team leader performs to keep a glass wall up to date. Objective data shared openly among all team members eliminates the finger pointing that often leads to position statements and conflict. With data, interests become clear and collaborative problem solving can take place.

When you focus on interests in negotiations, you can view the other person as a partner in problem solving. Because you are dealing with an interest, rather than a hard-line position, you and your partner can generate options for a mutually acceptable solution. The negotiation then becomes a problem-solving exercise and the potential for relationship-damaging conflict is removed.

This approach works especially well for Lean leaders who do not have positional authority over the people on the team. In that case, negotiation toward a solution becomes critical because you must accomplish a goal through people who do not report to you.

> Children's QDM director Stephanie Lenzner also notes that part of executive leadership is knowing how to tailor communication to best meet the needs of the audience. For example, Terry Schwartz knew the personal preferences of each doctor and used them. For one, the best method was to go through the secretary; for another, e-mail was the quickest and most effective method. Having to customize the communication for each doctor made it harder, but the payoff was the buy-in she got from the doctors— especially in an environment in which she has minimal positional authority over the physicians.

Visibility

Visibility is absolutely essential to your success as a Lean leader. Simply put, visibility means showing up. It means being present for the workshops you expect the team to participate in, and having positive input in those workshops. It means following through with action items and advancing the Lean effort between workshops. Finally, it means being willing to be the "face of Lean" for your clinic and using your personal credibility to drive the Lean transformation.

In some cases, a manager who is assigned responsibility for Lean will chose to delegate leadership of the effort, or worse yet hold the process hostage by not participating. Sometimes a dedicated team member will try to fill the void left by the absent manager. More often, though, frustration builds within the team, the manager loses credibility and respect, and the Lean effort becomes just another failed initiative.

When you put yourself at the forefront of the change process, the team understands the commitment you have made and will be more willing to follow your example. For example, Terry Schwartz at Children's Hospital of Wisconsin tells the story of transitioning the Orthopedic Center to the use of the patient status board. Some team members had a harder time than others adjusting to the use of the board and the need to continually move the magnets as patients progressed through the clinic. She took a highly visible approach and stood next to the status board all day to be sure it was being used. That investment of her time and personal credibility communicated clearly to the team that the board was important. The team not only adopted it, but has continued to evolve and improve its use.

Feedback

Providing feedback and recognition is a basic managerial skill that helps keep the team motivated and engaged during a Lean transformation.

In general, positive feedback and recognition are good ideas when you manage a work group or lead a project team. It is even more critical during a Lean transformation, because often the project team must go beyond their normal job requirements to complete extra work such as data collection or the creation of standard work. Further, a Lean transformation requires that people change the way they do their work, which can be stressful and emotional for some team members.

In those circumstances, the team needs to know that you appreciate their effort. Positive feedback and recognition are easy ways to show that appreciation.

Positive feedback is the informal, day-to-day message of "Thank you" or "Good job." In order to be most effective, positive feedback should follow these guidelines:

- It should be *timely*: Offer positive feedback right away; do not wait or the appropriate moment for the message will have passed.

- It should be *specific*: Although "Good job" is better than nothing, the feedback you offer should clearly state what was good and why. For example, "Thank you for staying late last night to finish those standard work documents. Without your extra effort, our workshop today could never have made so much progress."

- It should be *sincere*: People know intuitively when you are not sincere, and you will lose credibility with the team if you give positive feedback insincerely or for work that is part of the normal job.

Beyond the important day-to-day feedback, a Lean transformation offers lots of opportunities for recognition. Be creative in looking for ways to keep the team motivated. Sometimes a free lunch is appropriate; more often, recognition in the form of job enrichment is effective and lasting. For example, there may be opportunities for members of the Lean team to speak to senior leaders, providing exposure in the organization, or opportunities to work on special projects that result from the Lean initiative. Some healthcare systems have formal leadership development programs; for those that do not, participation on a Lean project team or an opportunity to present the Lean work are in themselves forms of recognition.

Strategic thinking

Strategic thinking is the ability to envision a future state and a plan to achieve it. It requires you to think several steps ahead, to understand today's workshop as the foundation of tomorrow's changes, and to see the logical progression of steps from the current state to the ideal.

In a Lean transformation, the Lean leader must think strategically in two fundamental areas: the flow of changes leading to the future state, and the organizational support needed to make those changes happen.

Achieving the future state

The primary tool available to the Lean leader in the first area is value stream mapping. Both the current state map and the future state map provide a powerful visual image of what changes are needed and help illustrate how the changes impact the overall system. By thoroughly completing the mapping exercises, you can develop a workable strategic action plan.

But even with that high-level plan, in your role as Lean leader you will encounter situations in which there is more than one solution to a given problem or change scenario and you will have to decide which direction the team will take. As a leader, your job is to take the team's input and come up with a direction in each workshop that makes sense in the context of the overall plan and Lean principles. It is important to let the team conduct trials and quick experiments with the solutions it generates, but ultimately you must have a plan and decide how the team will proceed. Without that responsibility clearly falling to one person (you), the team will flounder and progress will be slow.

Organizational support

Thinking strategically about organizational support means identifying champions who will help make change happen. The first champion you must identify is a physician in the clinic who is willing to implement

Lean. This physician champion will be someone you can work with, someone who will take direction and compromise when necessary, and someone who is willing to be personally involved with the Lean initiative. Avoid those physicians who want to delegate involvement and those who have such strong personalities that they will not work well as part of a team. An appropriate physician champion's team is probably already aligned with his or her way of thinking; they may make good core team members as well.

As you are identifying your physician champion, it is unwise to become too invested with the naysayers. In any clinic there will be people who oppose involvement with Lean (or any other improvement process); if there are too many naysayers, spend your time and effort elsewhere, rather than trying to convert them.

In addition to designating the physician champion, you must also communicate effectively with a respected medical leader about your Lean transformation and the successes and conflicts you encounter. By doing so, you help that person become a champion for Lean and you create an ally who can help remove roadblocks or resolve problems down the road.

Obtaining organizational support for your Lean effort means getting out and talking with the stakeholders involved: the physician champion, a respected medical leader, the project team members, and the rest of the clinic staff. You must identify the various interests these stakeholders have in the Lean project and focus on these interests in your communications (and negotiations). Building relationships and support in the organization cannot be accomplished solely using e-mail; make the effort to talk face-to-face. Then, when you encounter difficulties, you will have a network of supportive resources to help keep your Lean initiative going.

> "The most important thing hospital administrators can do to enhance their relationships with physicians is to respond to their needs and ideas... One way the administration can build its relationships with physicians is to make it easier for doctors to care for their patients. One of the top national priorities for hospitals, from the physician's perspective, is to make it easier to provide quality care for patients."
>
> From the *2007 Hospital Check-Up Report—Physician Perspectives on American Hospitals*, published by Press Ganey Associates, Inc, 2007

Long-term perspective

As we discussed in Chapter 1, we approach Lean one doctor at a time. That approach to implementation requires a long-term perspective. In this context, having a long-term perspective means being willing to take small steps in order to build competency and make progress in a controlled and planned way.

The task in front of you is potentially very large. A "clinic" may mean that there are several physicians holding specialized clinics on different days of the week, or even different parts of the day. The staff may change from day to day and from physician to physician; your clinic may even have multiple locations. The complexity in most healthcare systems makes it necessary to start Lean with a controlled scope—one doctor—but with an eye on the long-term goal of transforming the organization.

That one doctor's practice or clinic becomes the learning lab in which you will hone your skills and your approach to Lean, and from which you will expand to include other physicians and practices. It is important to recognize that the expansion might come as much as 18 months down the road, and plan the activity accordingly. Remember: Just as you would not begin a marathon with a sprint, do not start your Lean work with unsustainable resource use and fanfare.

Communicating with executives

As you lead your Lean project, communicate upward in the organization about problems you encounter, resources you need, and results you achieve. Communicating with executive management provides a great opportunity to generate visibility for your project, gain valuable presentation experience, and perhaps even boost your career.

One of the most important considerations related to executive communication is knowing when to initiate a discussion or presentation. In the face of problems or needed resources: Exhaust all other avenues before bring something to the attention of senior leadership. Use problem-solving techniques with your team to resolve the issue and involve your immediate manager and the managers of any other areas associated with the problem.

For reporting results: Wait until you have concrete, measurable, numeric results to report. Do not simply report activities such as workshops or training sessions; these do not take the place of bottom line results. Reporting that "We trained 40 people" or "We conducted four workshops" says to the executive that you have consumed resources without any return on that investment. Instead, set your goals at the beginning of the Lean project with a measurable business objective (for example, "We will increase capacity by 10 percent" or "We will reduce patient wait times by 25 percent") and present to the executive team only when you can demonstrate tangible progress.

Waiting until you have actual results before presenting your Lean efforts has the added benefit of building credibility with your audience. Something already accomplished is always more impressive than something you merely plan to do.

When you are speaking with executives or preparing a written document, remember that a busy executive is bombarded with information; your message must be clear and concise in order to be heard. He or she will not want to see pages of raw data or hear lengthy narratives about the process the team went through. A bottom line number, however, will make your point very clearly. If you feel compelled to bring research or data along to the meeting, keep it tucked away and present it only if a question is raised about your numbers or process.

When you bring a problem to an executive, it is a good idea to also bring along a solution or at least one or two well thought-out suggestions. If the executive is a hard-charging driver who makes quick decisions, bring along your best suggestion for solving the problem and come to a resolution in the meeting. However, if the executive is a thoughtful, analytical, data-driven type, you will want to provide relevant data, alternatives for resolving the problem, and some time to think about it. Understanding your audience will help you match the message to the personality and increase your chances of coming away with the results you want.

DEVELOPING YOUR LEADERSHIP SKILLS

It is not realistic to expect that you can concentrate on the fundamentals of Lean, the six success steps, and the leadership competencies at the same time. That's an overwhelming task. So do a quick self-assessment. About which of the leadership competencies do you feel the most confident? Which ones are your biggest opportunities for development? Prioritize the top two competencies for development and start there.

Leadership is notoriously difficult to teach and there is no magic solution. However, we have compiled some suggestions for developing your skills. Remember, do not try to develop all of these skills at once; create an action plan for yourself by selecting one or two skills to work on and trying the suggestions.

Negotiation

- Read *Getting to Yes* by Roger Fisher and William Ury.
- Volunteer to be part of (or lead) a problem-solving effort with another department. Be sure the team generates many alternatives before deciding on a solution to implement.

- Practice listening for positions and interests when you are in discussions with family and friends. When you hear a position, probe to find out the underlying interest; take note of the effect focusing on interests has on the conversation.

Visibility

- Walk around the clinic in which you will be leading Lean. Introduce yourself. If you do not know the staff, talk to everyone and learn their names.
- Practice "single-tasking" in all meetings and events. Let the team see you focusing on the matter at hand.
- Volunteer for—and complete—a highly visible action item in your next team meeting.

Recognition

- Practice offering positive feedback both at work and at home, until it no longer feels awkward to do so. Each time you offer positive feedback, make it sincere and specific.
- Offer positive feedback to strangers such as the parking attendant or the cashier at the grocery store. Note how your feedback changes the person's demeanor or motivation.
- Find out what your team considers a valued reward for future planning.

Strategic Thinking

- Learn to play chess or such games as Mastermind or Othello. Practice thinking two or three moves ahead (and see whether you can beat your kids!).
- Identify a physician champion based on the criteria in this section. Discuss your selection with a manager or trusted advisor, and plan to approach the physician with the opportunity to become involved with Lean.
- Read the Harvard Business Review article, *How Successful Leaders Think.*
- Create a backup plan for your Lean work in case your first choice for a physician champion is not successful.

Long-term Perspective

- Participate in value stream mapping with your clinic and develop a future state map.

- Walk through the future state value stream map and list the main changes the team has suggested. Lay out a tentative series of workshops needed to achieve the future state and estimate the time needed to accomplish those workshops. Communicate the length of the Lean journey to the team to help foster a long-term perspective.

- Set long-term goals in your personal life (like losing weight or learning another language). Outline the steps needed to achieve those goals and set a deadline.

- Plant a tree or grow tomatoes from seed. (Do this with children to practice explaining why things take so long.)

Communicating with Executives

- Develop a mentor relationship with an executive or leader in the organization. Ask this person for advice on presentations and other communication; ask to rehearse or review communications before delivering them.

- Look for opportunities to get in front of an executive audience, either at work or through volunteer activities or professional groups. Prepare ahead of time, and ask for coaching from a boss or mentor in the organization.

- Read communications coming from your organization's executives. Note the style and level of detail included, and try to mirror it in your own executive communication.

Epilogue: Where We Are Now?

Throughout this book, I've been telling you the story of my work with Children's Hospital of Wisconsin, transforming the Orthopedic Center with Lean principles. Now it seems time to present the end of the story, but at this point there is no end. There are two reasons.

The work we started at Children's continues because the program continues to grow as the word of great service, along with new offerings such as Sports Medicine, spreads around in the community. The entire team continues applying Lean in order to optimize physician schedules throughout the week, bring new physicians on-board, and grow the abilities of nurse practitioners and physician's assistants to see patients with specific diagnoses.

Second, the work continues because a culture change took place. With their new knowledge and toolset, the team focused its everyday efforts on improving patient service and improving processes while strengthening the Lean system. The Orthopedic team didn't just 'do Lean' and check it off the list. It has become part of the Orthopedic Center's operating system; it is just how everyone works. As Dr. Tassone said: "We can't imagine doing things any other way."

This is no different than how the system developed at Toyota. The relentless pursuit of perfection led Toyota to try solutions over decades, solutions that eventually became the Toyota Production System.

"Physicians now enjoy a moment of tactical advantage in the evolution of the struggle for control over healthcare in the United States. We suggest that the most effective way to capitalize on this—perhaps fleeting—position and to more permanently alter the balance of power in their favor is for physicians to establish strong and visionary leadership in healthcare quality improvement, with the goal of achieving unprecedented levels of excellence. Such an undertaking, if successful, could place the

> very essence of healthcare—defining, measuring, and improving its quality—in the hands of physicians."
>
> From Elise C. Becher, MD, MA, and Mark R. Chassin, MD, MPP, MPH. *Taking Healthcare Back: The Physician's Role in Quality Improvement*, Academic Medicine, Vol. 77, No. 10, October 2002.

An interesting outcome that we experienced but didn't anticipate is that when some of the ongoing problems were solved (for example, communication, duplication, or role confusion), new more transformative challenges surfaced. This second wave of problems, or opportunities, is provocative. The challenges get at the heart of what matters to doctors in particular and to healthcare workers in general: What impact can I have beyond providing care? Can I fundamentally change how I manage my practice to become a leader in the eyes of my team and my patients? Can I fundamentally transform myself? That's a question for another book.

The work has also expanded at Children's Hospital of Wisconsin. The six success steps, slightly translated, are relevant to the emergency departments, operating rooms, intensive care units, labs, radiology, pharmacy, materials distribution, and a variety of other types of outpatient clinics.

Think about how Lean applies in so many high-stakes healthcare environments. For instance, Maryanne Kessel, RN, MBA, the director of the Herma Heart Center at Children's Hospital, notes: "Pediatric cardiac healthcare is routinely a high-intensity and stressful environment where the lives of children are at risk with nearly every decision. This results in emotionally charged interactions around how the care is delivered."

Lean, she says, has allowed the staff some distance from that emotion as they evaluate processes. In her words: "Lean has allowed our program to step back form those less-than-productive emotional interactions and look at process improvement in a methodical, data-driven fashion. Lean has successfully placed the focus on how to make the patient's experience the best and safest care we can provide."

And there are other, data-driven reasons for applying and continuing Lean. In the Pediatric Intensive Care Unit, for example, Dr. Tom Rice, medical director of critical care, notes that a key motivator for transforming processes is that it also makes collecting solid, research-driven data more possible.

As he notes: "In the ICU, we're often dealing with rare events. And the evidence for taking care of such patients is essentially non-existent.... A lot may be based simply on what our individual experiences have been—and we may have only seen one similar case. So you can see, hospitals need to share this information with each other. We need to have ways to share what others have seen. And in order for this to happen in any sort of solid, evidence-based fashion, we need clearly-defined and workable processes."

On yet another front, application of Lean to business processes such as scheduling, invoicing, accounting, finance, marketing, and other processes is also in the works. As the understanding and confidence with Lean grows, the organization is beginning to set goals for strategic and critical areas to prioritize the focus with Lean resources. Frequent sharing of Lean solutions inside the organization has also resulted in leaders in each area examining their own challenges with a different set of glasses and trying new approaches.

We reached and still are reaching all the people we would have if we had begun with a massive training effort. But this way, when we get to new areas, people are waiting and asking to be involved.

Lean has perhaps opened the door for other methodologies, invented in other industries, to be tested in healthcare to solve problems and challenges. For example, there is an opportunity to examine processes with Lean and Six Sigma together. Six Sigma is a highly sophisticated problem solving methodology. Before deployment of a Six Sigma project, it is important to ask this question: Can I solve the problem through PDSA (Plan Do Study Act) cycle, 5 Why's, or any other traditional quality problem-solving techniques? If a project requires Six Sigma, then it is important to correctly scope and resource the effort.

An example of combining Lean and Six Sigma in our Orthopedic Center is examining how many follow-up visits particular types of patients need. After a new patient gets a cast, follow-up visits ensure proper healing. Researching historical data related to a particular diagnosis and then combining it with the knowledge and experience of the team can result in a set of guidelines for all providers to follow. Not only will this result in optimal use of provider time; it also will standardize certain aspects of care or create new protocols.

Clearly, Lean has the potential to transform healthcare—one doctor, one clinic, one hospital at a time. Visionaries within the field will continue to tap its potential and creatively adapt its principles, just as the power of Lean grew and expanded within the manufacturing and service sectors.

"I used to think of Lean as something that was used in the business world, not healthcare. Now, I know that it's useful in healthcare, too," says Dr. Theresa Mikhailov, of the Children's Hospital Pediatric Intensive Care Unit, where a Lean transformation is already underway.

"Lean is a methodology that helps healthcare providers take better care of patients, and ultimately, that is why we are all here."

Appendix A:
Introduction to Lean

A BRIEF AND SIMPLE HISTORY OF LEAN

Lean Manufacturing. Toyota Production System. Lean Enterprise. These names all refer to the same thing: the extraordinarily successful system for everything from manufacturing to research and development that Toyota has created over the past 50 years.

The history of Toyota's entrance into the American car market in a meaningful way is well known, so I'll give you the abridged version. The oil crisis of 1973 made many American consumers change their minds about large sedans and even larger, gas-guzzling engines. But American car manufacturers did not have high-quality, attractive small cars in their pipelines; in fact, they had years' worth of big cars and family sedans in their supply chains. When customer demands changed almost overnight, the American auto industry was not poised to adapt quickly.

Toyota, however, did adapt quickly. Toyota had developed a much shorter lead time, largely because of the environment in which they were operating in Japan. They did not have the square miles of storage space for manufactured (but not sold) vehicles that their American counterparts had, nor did they have the seemingly limitless supply of raw materials. Under the leadership of Taiichi Ohno, they had developed a system designed for efficiency, low inventory, and the flow of products directly to their customers rather than to warehouses and parking lots. This gave them a distinct advantage in a market in which customer requirements suddenly underwent a seismic shift.

The American auto manufacturers were challenged to introduce smaller, more fuel-efficient cars that people would actually buy, but their lots and dealerships were filled with large cars designed without attention to gas mileage and small cars built for the low end of the market. Consumers turned away from big cars, leaving the auto companies to carry the cost of that inventory while their market share dropped and giving Toyota a slice of the American market they have never given back.

DEPARTMENTS OR CELLS?

The rest of American manufacturing operates by and large using the same model used by the American auto industry: a departmental structure with supervisors who direct the work of the front-line workers in each of those departments. Departments provide a logical structure, but lead to a host of problems well known in the manufacturing world: departmental schedules that are mismatched and lead ironically to both material shortages and excess inventories, transportation of material between departments, waiting, rework, and a focus on internal department goals rather than on external customer requirements.

That's certainly the world I found when I began my career in manufacturing. The department I joined as a chemical engineer out of college was not just isolated from the other departments in the plant, it was a separate building. It may as well have been a separate country. I took the communication challenges and scheduling frustrations as part and parcel of manufacturing—and even learned to thrive in that environment—until I had the opportunity to work in a cell.

That cell was unique in the company. It made one product family from beginning to end: It received the raw materials, made the product, packaged it, and shipped it without separate receiving, production, and shipping departments. With no departments, there was only one schedule. There was a small team of engineers and operators all located in the same space and all focused on the same goal. When there was a problem, everyone was present and able to voice opinions and lend expertise. The team knew how they were performing against the customer-driven goals because performance data was posted in the cell area. The team consistently out-performed other areas of the plant. Wouldn't it be great, I thought, if every manufacturing area worked like this?

When I later studied Lean, I recognized some of the same principles. Toyota is organized in product-focused cells, rather than in departments. Each cell is self-contained, and runs as a "mini-business." The mini-business concept means that each cell has customer-focused goals as well as quality improvement goals, and manages its work accordingly. The team leader is responsible for the cell's performance and works to support the front line operators to be sure they have everything they need to accomplish those goals. The team leader tracks performance data, makes sure that raw materials are stocked, and fills in for absences—quite a departure from the traditional supervisor.

The focus of a cell is on the front-line operators and the work they do. Compare this approach to a traditional American manufacturing company with its emphasis on executives and an often contentious relationship with front line workers. In fact, at Toyota managers and executives must spend years working on the front lines as part of their career path; even the pay differential between the assembly line and the executive suite reflects this cooperative approach.

LEAN OUTSIDE OF THE MANUFACTURING WORLD

Interest in and knowledge of the Toyota Production System (TPS) grew and became branded as Lean (thanks to researchers James Womack and Daniel Jones). Books like Womack and Jones' *The Machine that Changed the World* brought Lean to an even wider audience in 1990, and the concepts and tools found their way into other industries. First, they spread to manufacturing outside of automotive. In my career, I've had the opportunity to apply Lean thinking to paint and chemical manufacturing and even the building of yachts. Within a decade, adventurous Lean practitioners were applying Lean to service industries and office environments and to functions such as research and development. I've worked with computer designers and researchers creating new helicopters to achieve flow, not of products or even services but of knowledge.

Healthcare organizations recognized that Lean had something for them as well around the turn of the century. Lean dovetails nicely with other quality initiatives in healthcare, such as the "Transforming Care at the Bedside" nursing initiative sponsored by the Robert Wood Johnson Foundation. But through its many evolutions, Lean is at risk of becoming like so many other quality systems in the US—something external and artificial superimposed on organizations that glom onto tools and techniques and miss the all-important *whole*. There are indeed tools and techniques in Lean and this book describes how they work in healthcare. But Lean is truly a different approach because the whole is greater than the sum of its parts.

In Appendix B we'll take a look at the types of waste that Lean removes and define common terms in a Lean system. What's harder to outline so succinctly is the philosophy that makes it all work—that the people doing the jobs are the ones who know the most about it, that an engineer's or executive's or physician's opinion is no more important than that of the front-line worker or nurse or orderly. And that breaking down barriers—whether departmental walls or barriers of rank, education, or access to information—is the prerequisite for improving flow. So study the tools and techniques by all means, but remember that true transformation means seeing the whole.

Appendix B: Glossary and Explanations of Lean Principles and Terms

FLOW, VALUE, AND WASTE

Flow in the Lean sense is a manufacturing term. It refers to the ideal state of product moving through a manufacturing process without stopping.

Wherever the product stops, it piles up, gets stacked in aisles, gets lost or damaged, and hides system-level problems in a sea of inventory. The goal is to keep the product moving, which requires that the system be completely focused on the product, make that product according to the rate of customer demand, and resolve problems immediately as they occur. Every step in the journey of meeting that goal has huge implications—and often requires huge changes—for the manufacturing system.

In healthcare, and specifically for the clinic, that product is the patient. In an ideal state, the patient would enter the clinic and move continuously from check-in to check-out without stopping. Each time the patient stops, the wait time is indicative of a larger issue with the system. A wait at Radiology, for example, may indicate that the department is short of staff, that equipment is not working, or that the radiology resources are mismatched with patient schedules or needs. A wait for the physician once the patient is in the exam room may indicate that the physician is overloaded with other demands that do not fit into the schedule, or that the clinic is chronically overbooked. A wait at a supporting department may mean that the workload is not balanced and that department experiences work in waves that cause delays.

VALUE-ADDED ACTIVITY

Across industries in manufacturing, a typical operator spends no more than 25 percent of his or her time on *value-added activities*—activities that actually change the product and are valued by the customer. The rest of the workday is spent dealing with waste: walking to retrieve supplies that are too far away, trying to find the right parts at the right time, waiting for a shared resource such as a fork truck or a common press, or fixing defects, to name a few. When manufacturing firms focus on removing the waste from the operator's job so more time can be spent on value-added tasks related to the product, they see substantial productivity increases.

The same scenario is true of physicians. The value-added time is the time spent with the patient, yet that adds up to only minutes of the total hours the physician typically spends in the clinic. Physicians experience the same wastes: missing paperwork, patients who are not roomed in a timely fashion, incorrect x-rays, having to walk long distances within the clinic to see patients or retrieve information from remote terminals in work rooms, waiting to get more information from referring physicians, or patients who are scheduled in the wrong clinic by a central scheduling function.

WASTE

The Toyota Production System identifies several primary types of waste that are typically present in any process or system, regardless of the product being produced or the service provided.

Overproduction

Overproduction is the primary waste in any system and it causes a host of other problems. Overproduction means making more of a particular product than the next step in the system can use. This next step in the system can be an internal step (for example, producing more of a sub-assembled part than the next station in a manufacturing process can use) or an external step (for example, producing more cars than can be sold). That extra inventory sits around, gets stacked in the aisles, gets damaged or lost, and creates added expenses.

In healthcare, that extra inventory takes on a very personal face. Overproduction may mean that one part of the process goes quickly and causes a backlog of patients waiting at the next step. Those waiting patients become frustrated and have a lower overall satisfaction with their experience in the healthcare facility. Because overproduction is both a waste in and of itself and a symptom of other problems within the healthcare system, patients waiting in the process is a flag indicating that improvements are needed. It's interesting to note that pull systems and kanban work as well in healthcare as they do in manufacturing; although the "product" is people and their healthcare, the principles of designing efficient processes remain the same.

Inventory

The big problem with inventory in any system is either having too much of it on hand so that it becomes hard to store and manage or not having the right items on hand when they are needed.

Both of these problems are prevalent in healthcare, most obviously in inventories of supplies. Excessive levels of supplies are often stored where convenient and are sometimes hard to find. They become obsolete and have to be moved or replaced, which takes time from other value-added tasks that staff must accomplish. Carrying inventory also makes tracing the source of quality problems difficult, because suppliers are not notified in a timely fashion of problems with materials. The lack of the right supplies in the right locations can compromise patient care.

Defects

Defects are an easily understood source of waste in the process. Some defects can be corrected with time and resources; others require that the product be discarded, resulting in a waste of time and materials.

In healthcare, defects are mistakes. Mistakes can occur for a number of reasons such as a chaotic work environment, duplicate paperwork, poor communication, and poorly defined processes and roles, among others.

Lean provides tools such as standard work and error proofing to create systems that eliminate the possibility of errors and defects. In fact, the more critical the work, the more indispensable error proofing and standard work become. Lean believes that to err is human, but to let that error turn into a defect is a failure of the system in place.

Motion

Motion refers to the movement of people in the course of doing their jobs. Unnecessary motion wastes time and energy and may contribute to ergonomic issues in the workplace. Wasted motion results when a worker must walk a long distance to use a piece of equipment or collect tools. It results when a workstation is not properly organized and the worker must search for what he needs to perform the work. Motion improves when a department structure is broken down into a cell structure organized around the steps in the process, allowing the process to flow.

Once the staff begins to evaluate how far they travel for forms and supplies, for example, decisions about relocating items within the facility become easy. Workplace organization, or 5S, becomes a critical tool to reduce wasted staff motion; it results in higher staff satisfaction and a less stressful work environment.

Additionally, focusing on patient and staff movement within the facility can have a dramatic effect on patient wait times and family satisfaction, staff communication and handoffs, and resource levels and efficiencies. Evaluating wasted motion has big implications for the physical layout of the facility as well.

Over Processing

Over processing refers to wasted steps in the process—steps that may be redundant or performed simply because that's the way it has always been done. Patient paperwork is a good example of over processing in healthcare. The same information is gathered in several places, leaving the patient with the impression that various functions within the healthcare facility do not communicate with each other, and increasing patient frustration. From the customer (patient) perspective, that repetitive gathering of information without an agreed upon plan is over processing.

The lack of clear roles and processes can also result in over processing. For example, several members of the clinic staff could ask the same questions of the patient without a plan for communicating with each other. This not only leads to extra steps for the staff, but adds to patient frustration as well.

Transportation

Transportation refers to wasted movement of equipment. This causes both wasted staff motion and potential damage to equipment.

A good example of equipment movement in healthcare occurs in the operating room. Specialized equipment that is used frequently is sometimes stored far away from the point of use, causing delays in room turnovers and patient processes.

Waiting

This waste occurs when a value-added operator waits to complete a process step for any reason: parts coming from a warehouse, missing supplies, confusion about what to do next, the need for approval from a supervisor, or a lack of available equipment. This waste has implications for workspace design and facilities design. It supports organization location and access.

In healthcare, waiting is a major opportunity for improvement. Evaluating this waste further helps us understand the workload and balance of resources in a given area. A physician waiting for a patient to be roomed, a nurse waiting for a physician's assistant, and a casting technician waiting for clarification are all opportunities to identify better handoffs and balance resources and tasks.

GLOSSARY OF LEAN TERMS

5S

5S is the Japanese-developed method for evaluating and improving workplace organization:

- Sort: separating the necessary from the unnecessary items in the workplace and clearing out the clutter.

- Stabilize: organizing what's left so that it is readily accessible to the person doing the job.

- Shine: cleaning everything to promote pride and attention to environment.

- Standardize: maintaining the changes through formal job responsibilities and policy.

- Sustain: placing a long-term emphasis on organization and improvement.

Cell

A cell is a small group of functions located in the same space in order to provide a specific care process most efficiently. For example, a fractures clinic in Orthopedics would create a cell by co-locating radiology, physical therapy, and casting in the same space as the exam rooms. Creating the cell eliminates the wastes of motion and waiting for the patient and dramatically improves communication and efficiency for the staff.

Changeover

Changeover is the period of time between the end of one process and the beginning of the next. For example, changeover in a clinic setting starts when the physician finishes with one patient's exam and ends with the start of the next patient's exam. All of the activities that take place outside of the physician's consultation—for example, cleaning the exam room, setting up for the next patient, and so on—can be considered changeover.

External Changeover

Steps in the changeover process are external if they occur when the "machine" is running and producing a value-added product—when the physician or other care provider is seeing another patient. The team can achieve patient flow when as many of the changeover steps as possible are made external and the physician can move from exam room to exam room.

FIFO Lane

FIFO stands for "First In First Out." It is a way of controlling how many patients are in a system at any one time. A FIFO lane is similar to ping-pong balls in a tube: only so many fit, and no more. When the FIFO lane is filled, no more patients can be accommodated until there is room in the system. The patients currently in the system are seen and cared for in the order in which they were added. FIFO lanes are simple ways to ensure that the level schedule stays level and patients are seen in order.

Flow

Flow refers to an ideal state in which the person or thing moving through the process never stops to wait for the next process step.

Glass Wall

The term glass wall refers to an area visible to all team members in which data about performance metrics is posted. Typically the team leader collects the data after the team decides which performance metrics are most important. This data helps level the playing field for problem solving and process improvement input, as all team members have the same access to the same information.

Internal Changeover

Steps in the changeover process are internal if they occur when the "machine" is not running—when the physician or other care provider is not with another patient. The goal of improving the changeover process is to reduce or eliminate internal changeover steps.

Kanban

A kanban is a signal that accompanies inventory in a pull system. A kanban may be a reorder form that is sent to a materials supplier, or any other signal that is passed between processes to indicate that more products (or people) can be placed into the system.

Level Schedule

A level schedule is one that balances types of work in a given workday. Level schedules are most often used in the context of scheduling templates that allow the team adequate time to see patients without falling behind schedule. Level schedules will vary based on the physician and type of patients seen. For example, in a busy fractures clinic, a level schedule may be one that places two follow-up patients in a row, and then one new patient.

Process Map

A process map is a tool that identifies the individual steps within a particular process. Process mapping is used to break a single process into its steps and analyze opportunities for improvement.

Pull System

A pull system is one in which each process produces only what the next step in the process needs, and no more. Pull systems are the next best thing to achieving true flow in a Lean system. In pull systems, each process step "tells" its supplying process to produce or send more. For example, using a pull system to reorder supplies would mean that supplies are only replenished when they reach a predetermined order point.

Push System

A push system is one in which each step produces its product without regard for the needs of the next step in the process. Push systems typically result in the wastes of waiting, overproduction, inventory, motion, and transportation as extra materials must be moved and stored, or as patients experience long wait times.

Shared Resource

A shared resource is one specialized person or piece of equipment that many staff members or patients need. The physician is the shared resource in the clinic or practice. A shared resource is a potential pacemaker in the process, which means that special attention must be paid to how that shared resources' time is scheduled.

Spaghetti Diagram

A spaghetti diagram is a picture of the movement involved in the completion of a given process. Spaghetti diagrams are made by watching a person complete a task with a rough sketch of the workspace in hand. Each time the person being observed moves, walks to get something, or reaches for a form, the person drawing the map makes a line indicating that movement. Spaghetti diagrams illustrate waste of movement and prompt rethinking about how workspaces are designed.

Standard Work

Standard work is a document that defines one person's role in a particular task. Standard work documents list the main process steps, details of those steps where needed, the time it takes to complete those steps, and a diagram of the workspace's physical layout.

Supermarket

A supermarket is a controlled level of inventory that is kept between process steps in a pull system. When that inventory is needed, it is pulled from the supermarket. When the supermarket must be replenished, a signal (kanban) is sent to the supplying process to produce or send more. Supermarkets are a critical concept for moving frequently used items to the point of use, and for efficiently managing inventories of forms and supplies.

Team Leader

A team leader is one member of the clinic or practice staff—usually a nurse—who is specifically responsible for patient flow through the care processes. The team leader is in charge of the patient status board and uses it to help direct the physician's workflow. The team leader also collects data for the glass wall and leads problem solving and improvement efforts for the team.

Value-Added Activity

Value-added activity is a step in any given process that changes the person or thing going through the process (filing or moving, for example, don't count) and about which the customer cares.

Value Stream Map

A value stream map is a 40,000-foot view of steps and processes required to fulfill patient needs. Looking at a value stream map is like taking the roof off of the building and looking down to identify where the patient receives care, and where the patient waits for the next step to occur. Value stream maps are critical in Lean implementations to see the entire care process as a cohesive whole and ensure that changes are not disjointed.

Visual Control

Visual control means communicating the status of all patient processes visually, so that anyone walking into the staff environment can tell which exam rooms are ready for the physician, where the patients are in the process, and whether or not the practice is on schedule. Sharing this status information—as well the process metrics posted on the glass wall—has important implications for team dynamics, as all team members have the same access to information.

Waste

Waste is any part of the process that consumes resources but provides no value. Lean is essentially the systematic and relentless focus on removing waste from the care process.

Appendix C:
Other Resources

Much has been written about Lean and its genesis at Toyota. Good resources include *Lean Thinking* by Dan Jones and James Womack and *Becoming Lean* by Jeffrey Liker. Steven Spear and Ken Bowen's *Harvard Business Review* article, "Decoding the DNA of the Toyota Production System" (1999), provides insight into some of the guiding philosophies of Lean. *Learning to See* by Mike Rother and John Shook is an excellent introduction to value stream mapping.

For those who want a deeper dive into Lean, we recommend *The New Manufacturing Challenge* and *Results from the Heart*, both by Kyoshi Suzaki, and *The Evolution of a Manufacturing System at Toyota*, by Takahiro Fujimoto.

Appendix D:
My Lean Background

I finished my BS in Chemical Engineering at Cleveland State University and joined PPG Industries as a chemical engineer, working at the resin plant in Oak Creek, Wisconsin, for four years before moving to technical service. Unlike at the resin plant, the tech service job forced me to get out in front of operators at customer plants to solve problems with paint application.

That job was really formative for me. I worked primarily with the overnight shift at Outboard Marine Co. in Calhoun, Georgia. There, because of my Indian heritage, I had to overcome racial stereotypes ("You're not from around here, are you?") and get the operators to work with me. I learned to listen carefully to operator input, and not assume that because I was the college-educated engineer that I knew everything. Even though I tend to have a naturally accommodating and polite style, this third-shift work at Outboard Marine certainly helped me refine my interpersonal skills. (And I learned that a box of doughnuts sometimes goes farther than an MBA when it comes to making changes with the front-line operators!) I solved some technically difficult problems and received some organizational attention with the Coatings division of PPG.

The main lesson I learned: The key is to work *with* operators to implement changes when you have no positional authority. Collaboration and an understanding attitude are key.

From there, I came back to the Oak Creek plant as a business manager for the Cationic product line—a well-established and important line for PPG. The problems I encountered there were ones of capacity: PPG could sell all the Cationic coatings it could produce, but the line had some quality issues that limited its production. I was chosen to be trained as a Six Sigma Blackbelt at the Whirlpool Corporation (one of the line's main customers) to help solve those problems. I found myself truly in my element: my wife says I took to Six Sigma like a fish to water. At any rate,

I successfully applied the methodology to the Cationic line. I also learned to manage people through this assignment, as I had a team that needed some re-energizing. I was able to use some of the collaborative style I developed through my stint as a technical service rep to get the Cationic team fully engaged in the improvement process. I completed my MBA during this time as well.

> **The main lesson I learned: Six Sigma problem-solving works in a variety of settings and provides important tools for improvement.**

I left the Cationic Business Manager position to relocate to Pittsburgh, where the position of Business Unit Improvement Catalyst was created at the Springdale coatings plant. There, I studied Lean manufacturing at the University of Michigan. But interestingly, none of the faculty at the Center for Professional Development seemed to have any guidance to offer about how Lean would apply to a process such as making paint. (They went on to use PPG as a case study later, but in 1999 had not yet thought very far outside of discreet parts manufacturing). I combined Lean and Six Sigma to re-imagine how paint is made. With the primary stakeholders for one product line, we created a future state vision for that line using value stream mapping. We spearheaded a Six Sigma project that solved the tough problems in implementing the future state, and the changes resulted in a huge reduction in the level of inventory needed for that product line. Springdale became the model line for the entire coatings division, and the manager of the line spent a lot of time giving tours to other paint plants. The project was executed in an understated way, with no fanfare and no communication about it until the results were achieved. That strategy worked well, especially in contrast to the approach of talking about plans and then falling short of delivering results.

> **The main lesson I learned: With some creativity, Lean Manufacturing principles could be applied outside of discreet parts manufacturing. Another key lesson for me: It's important to get consensus leading up to big changes.**

I left PPG after that project to work for one of the first of the online auction houses that shook up the B2B sourcing process. I started there as an account manager, and then moved into a role in which I was responsible for shortening the lead time from proposal to auction using Lean techniques. Using Lean in the world of paint manufacturing required "translating" a lot of the tools for continuous flow processes (making 5000 gallons of paint, versus making rear view windows or some other discreet products). But using Lean for auctions required a major translation. At times I felt I was pushing the boundaries of what Lean could do, and I learned in the process how to communicate manufacturing strategies to people in other businesses.

The main lesson I learned: It takes *lots* of creativity and strategizing, but Lean can be successfully applied to an "invisible" product line (or a service).

I later relocated to Florida and rejoined PPG at LYNX Services, a wholly-owned subsidiary that processed insurance claims about damaged windshields. My position there was created to apply Lean to the process of insurance claims. The company generated income by processing claims; it could improve its financial performance if it could increase capacity without adding to headcount. Again, I found myself translating the concepts of Lean for another industry—this one a service provided electronically. I remember one meeting with the quality team during which we divided a flipchart into two columns and wrote the manufacturing terms on one side, then looked for a parallel in the insurance claims side. That very literal translation made a lot of light bulbs go on—both for the LYNX team and for me: Lean applied everywhere.

The main lesson I learned: Lean applies to an even less tangible process—a service provided via electronic means.

I eventually left the insurance processing company to start a consulting firm, FlowOne. My first major client was a military helicopter maker in the Research & Development division. The goal was to shorten the time it took to develop new models while still meeting customer requirements. There, the process was messy and completely in the heads of engineers. I also began working with a yacht-building division, where I discovered that applying Lean to a product as large as a yacht means that the process has to move the thing (rather than the thing moving through the process). I developed a cell structure for yacht building (even though the product itself didn't "move" along any assembly line). Here I also worked intensely with the team leader role; implementing this proved to be a significant turning point for all of the plants.

The main lesson I learned: Lean can be applied to how knowledge is created and passed along in the design process. And a successful and deep application of Lean involves negotiation and consensus building.

Appendix E:
A3 Problem Solving Form

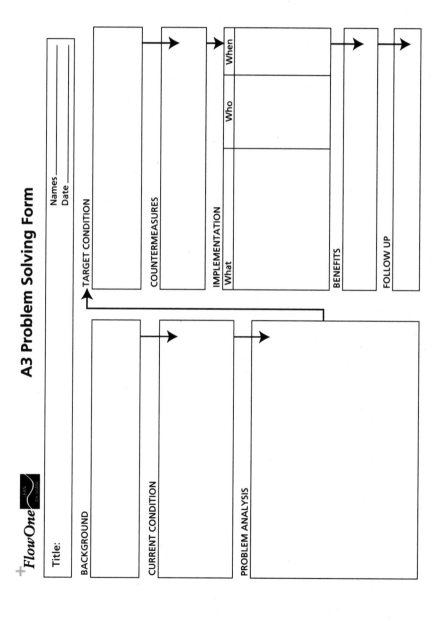

Index

Page numbers in *italics* refer to tables or illustrations.

Belong to the Quality Community!

Established in 1946, ASQ is a global community of quality experts in all fields and industries. ASQ is dedicated to the promotion and advancement of quality tools, principles, and practices in the workplace and in the community.

The Society also serves as an advocate for quality. Its members have informed and advised the U.S. Congress, government agencies, state legislatures, and other groups and individuals worldwide on quality-related topics.

Vision

By making quality a global priority, an organizational imperative, and a personal ethic, ASQ becomes the community of choice for everyone who seeks quality technology, concepts, or tools to improve themselves and their world.

ASQ is...

- More than 90,000 individuals and 700 companies in more than 100 countries

- The world's largest organization dedicated to promoting quality

- A community of professionals striving to bring quality to their work and their lives

- The administrator of the Malcolm Baldrige National Quality Award

- A supporter of quality in all sectors including manufacturing, service, healthcare, government, and education

- YOU

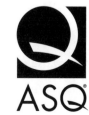

Visit www.asq.org for more information.

ASQ Membership

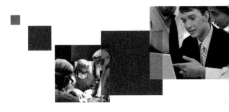

Research shows that people who join associations experience increased job satisfaction, earn more, and are generally happier.* ASQ membership can help you achieve this while providing the tools you need to be successful in your industry and to distinguish yourself from your competition. So why wouldn't you want to be a part of ASQ?

Networking

Have the opportunity to meet, communicate, and collaborate with your peers within the quality community through conferences and local ASQ section meetings, ASQ forums or divisions, ASQ Communities of Quality discussion boards, and more.

Professional Development

Access a wide variety of professional development tools such as books, training, and certifications at a discounted price. Also, ASQ certifications and the ASQ Career Center help enhance your quality knowledge and take your career to the next level.

Solutions

Find answers to all your quality problems, big and small, with ASQ's Knowledge Center, mentoring program, various e-newsletters, *Quality Progress* magazine, and industry-specific products.

Access to Information

Learn classic and current quality principles and theories in ASQ's Quality Information Center (QIC), *ASQ Weekly* e-newsletter, and product offerings.

Advocacy Programs

ASQ helps create a better community, government, and world through initiatives that include social responsibility, Washington advocacy, and Community Good Works.

Visit www.asq.org/membership for more information on ASQ membership.

*2008, The William E. Smith Institute for Association Research

ASQ Certification

ASQ certification is formal recognition by ASQ that an individual has demonstrated a proficiency within, and comprehension of, a specified body of knowledge at a point in time. Nearly 150,000 certifications have been issued. ASQ has members in more than 100 countries, in all industries, and in all cultures. ASQ certification is internationally accepted and recognized.

Benefits to the Individual

- New skills gained and proficiency upgraded
- Investment in your career
- Mark of technical excellence
- Assurance that you are current with emerging technologies
- Discriminator in the marketplace
- Certified professionals earn more than their uncertified counterparts
- Certification is endorsed by more than 125 companies

Benefits to the Organization

- Investment in the company's future
- Certified individuals can perfect and share new techniques in the workplace
- Certified staff are knowledgeable and able to assure product and service quality

Quality is a global concept. It spans borders, cultures, and languages. No matter what country your customers live in or what language they speak, they demand quality products and services. You and your organization also benefit from quality tools and practices. Acquire the knowledge to position yourself and your organization ahead of your competition.

Certifications Include

- Biomedical Auditor – CBA
- Calibration Technician – CCT
- HACCP Auditor – CHA
- Pharmaceutical GMP Professional – CPGP
- Quality Inspector – CQI
- Quality Auditor – CQA
- Quality Engineer – CQE
- Quality Improvement Associate – CQIA
- Quality Technician – CQT
- Quality Process Analyst – CQPA
- Reliability Engineer – CRE
- Six Sigma Black Belt – CSSBB
- Six Sigma Green Belt – CSSGB
- Software Quality Engineer – CSQE
- Manager of Quality/Organizational Excellence – CMQ/OE

Visit www.asq.org/certification to apply today!

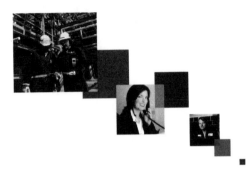

ASQ Training

Classroom-based Training

ASQ offers training in a traditional classroom setting on a variety of topics. Our instructors are quality experts and lead courses that range from one day to four weeks, in several different cities. Classroom-based training is designed to improve quality and your organization's bottom line. Benefit from quality experts; from comprehensive, cutting-edge information; and from peers eager to share their experiences.

Web-based Training

Virtual Courses

ASQ's virtual courses provide the same expert instructors, course materials, interaction with other students, and ability to earn CEUs and RUs as our classroom-based training, without the hassle and expenses of travel. Learn in the comfort of your own home or workplace. All you need is a computer with Internet access and a telephone.

Self-paced Online Programs

These online programs allow you to work at your own pace while obtaining the quality knowledge you need. Access them whenever it is convenient for you, accommodating your schedule.

Some Training Topics Include

- Auditing
- Basic Quality
- Engineering
- Education
- Healthcare
- Government
- Food Safety
- ISO
- Leadership
- Lean
- Quality Management
- Reliability
- Six Sigma
- Social Responsibility

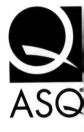

Visit www.asq.org/training for more information.